Aydogan Ozcan

NON-DESTRUCTIVE OPTICAL CHARACTERIZATION TOOLS

Aydogan Ozcan

NON-DESTRUCTIVE OPTICAL CHARACTERIZATION TOOLS

Spectral Interferometry Using Minimum-phase Functions

VDM Verlag Dr. Müller

Impressum/Imprint (nur für Deutschland/ only for Germany)
Bibliografische Information der Deutschen Nationalbibliothek: Die Deutsche Nationalbibliothek verzeichnet diese Publikation in der Deutschen Nationalbibliografie; detaillierte bibliografische Daten sind im Internet über http://dnb.d-nb.de abrufbar.
Alle in diesem Buch genannten Marken und Produktnamen unterliegen warenzeichen-, marken- oder patentrechtlichem Schutz bzw. sind Warenzeichen oder eingetragene Warenzeichen der jeweiligen Inhaber. Die Wiedergabe von Marken, Produktnamen, Gebrauchsnamen, Handelsnamen, Warenbezeichnungen u.s.w. in diesem Werk berechtigt auch ohne besondere Kennzeichnung nicht zu der Annahme, dass solche Namen im Sinne der Warenzeichen- und Markenschutzgesetzgebung als frei zu betrachten wären und daher von jedermann benutzt werden dürften.

Coverbild: www.purestockx.com

Verlag: VDM Verlag Dr. Müller Aktiengesellschaft & Co. KG
Dudweiler Landstr. 99, 66123 Saarbrücken, Deutschland
Telefon +49 681 9100-698, Telefax +49 681 9100-988, Email: info@vdm-verlag.de
Zugl.: Stanford, Stanford University, Diss., 2005

Herstellung in Deutschland:
Schaltungsdienst Lange o.H.G., Berlin
Books on Demand GmbH, Norderstedt
Reha GmbH, Saarbrücken
Amazon Distribution GmbH, Leipzig
ISBN: 978-3-639-10449-3

Imprint (only for USA, GB)
Bibliographic information published by the Deutsche Nationalbibliothek: The Deutsche Nationalbibliothek lists this publication in the Deutsche Nationalbibliografie; detailed bibliographic data are available in the Internet at http://dnb.d-nb.de.
Any brand names and product names mentioned in this book are subject to trademark, brand or patent protection and are trademarks or registered trademarks of their respective holders. The use of brand names, product names, common names, trade names, product descriptions etc. even without a particular marking in this works is in no way to be construed to mean that such names may be regarded as unrestricted in respect of trademark and brand protection legislation and could thus be used by anyone.

Cover image: www.purestockx.com

Publisher:
VDM Verlag Dr. Müller Aktiengesellschaft & Co. KG
Dudweiler Landstr. 99, 66123 Saarbrücken, Germany
Phone +49 681 9100-698, Fax +49 681 9100-988, Email: info@vdm-publishing.com
Copyright © 2008 VDM Verlag Dr. Müller Aktiengesellschaft & Co. KG and licensors
All rights reserved. Saarbrücken 2008

Printed in the U.S.A.
Printed in the U.K. by (see last page)
ISBN: 978-3-639-10449-3

ACKNOWLEDGMENTS

I not only use all of the brains I have, but all I can borrow.
Woodrow Wilson

It is close to the end of my fifth year here at Stanford… Only a few days to my graduation. As always is the case, time goes by, and as my father always said, "starting something is almost like finishing it". That view can only be truly understood at the end.

Stanford gave me all the great opportunities that a Ph.D. student should have. The excellence in research and education, combined with a beautiful climate and a wonderful neighborhood put Stanford way ahead of other top universities within USA. If I were given the chance to choose any university, without hesitation, Stanford would, once again, be my first choice.

I am grateful to many people who made my stay at Stanford a wonderful experience. My deepest gratitude goes due to my advisors, Gordon S. Kino and Michel J. F. Digonnet. They were involved in every aspect of my research, and were always available for a discussion. They were an inspiration for me on many issues, including how to run a research group. In terms of written and oral communication skills, they spend a great deal of their valuable time to pass a high level of quality to their students. And I am very grateful that they do; considering my own communication skills before I joined the group, thanks to their teachings, I can clearly see many positive changes. I wish to express my sincere gratitude to them for being such great advisors.

I am also grateful to Olav Solgaard for being an inspirational professor at Stanford and also for serving as a reader in my thesis committee. I took all the courses that he taught at Stanford between 2000 and 2004, and his style of teaching was truly inspirational. I learned most of my fundamental optics knowledge from his classes.

I want to also acknowledge my gratitude to Umran Inan for being the chair of my oral defense committee.

I also acknowledge my collaborators Feridun Ay and Atilla Aydinli of the Physics Department at Bilkent University. Beginning May 2004, we worked very closely with the Bilkent group on thermally poled germanosilicate thin film project. Their enthusiasm and excitement were a constant source of motivation for me. Also, on fiber Bragg grating characterization, I am grateful to David Pureur of Highwave Optical Technologies, Lannion, France for supplying the experimental data. On sub-picosecond pulse characterization, I am deeply thankful to David N. Fittinghoff of Lawrence Livermore National Laboratory and to Selcuk Akturk of Georgia Institute of Technology for their valuable discussions and for supplying the experimental raw data.

I would like to also deeply thank to our administrative associate Ann Guss. Her perfectionism in handling the administrative issues gave me a greater opportunity to focus on my research. I also thank to my lab mates Ueyn Block, Vinayak Dangui, Hyang Kyun Kim, and Stephane Blin, together with Utkan Demirci, Ali Kemal Okyay, Ragip Pala and all my friends for making it fun to be at Stanford. I am also grateful to our sponsor Litton Systems, Inc.

Last but definitely not least, I thank to my family for their continued support and patience.

DEDICATION

To all the greatest minds of the science community, aiming to make the world a better place to live in...

TABLE OF CONTENTS

i

LIST OF TABLES

LIST OF FIGURES

CHAPTER 1: INTRODUCTION

Somewhere, something incredible is waiting to be known.
Carl Sagan

This dissertation describes our contributions to the application of Fourier transform theory to retrieve vital information about various physical phenomena.[1-24] This introductory chapter begins with a brief discussion of Fourier transform theory and its impact on science and technology. Next, the significance of the Fourier transform phase and magnitude and their physical interpretation are discussed. Finally, the contributions and the organization of the dissertation are presented.

1.1 FOURIER TRANSFORM THEORY AND ITS IMPACT ON SCIENCE AND TECHNOLOGY

Beginning in the 19th century, Fourier transform theory, often referred to by mathematicians as harmonic analysis,[25] has played a huge role in the evolution of science and technology. Although it is widely used in today's world, the father of harmonic analysis, Baron Joseph Fourier, had enormous difficulty persuading the great mathematicians of his time such as Laplace, Lagrance, and Poisson of the significance of his analysis. His important memoir *"On the Propagation of Heat in Solid Bodies",* where he first introduced the concept of expansion of functions using trigonometric series (known today as the Fourier series), encountered significant resistance and numerous objections from nearly all the famous names of the world of mathematics in 1807. Fourier tried to address all these challenges, but was not fully successful. As pointed out in Ref. 26, *"All these (his answers) are written with such exemplary clarity - from a logical as opposed to calligraphic point of view - that their inability to persuade Laplace and Lagrange ... provides a good index of the originality of Fourier's views...".* Fourier was clearly well ahead of his time and the true groundbreaking extent of his analysis would be realized much later.

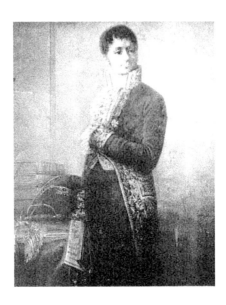

Fig. 1. Baron Joseph Fourier, the father of harmonic analysis; b. 1768, Auxerre, France, d. 1830, Paris, France.

It is interesting to note that today's mathematicians do not consider Fourier's work among the most significant theories in the history of mathematics. While most mathematicians consider Gauss to be the greatest mathematician of all time, Fourier does not even place among the top ten.[27-28] To an electrical engineer or an applied physicist, on the other hand, the legacy of Fourier is far more influential. What makes Joseph Fourier so special for engineers and physicist can be found in his famous quote: *"The profound study of nature is the most fertile source of mathematical discoveries."* The intuition that Fourier analysis brought to scientists and engineers had the same effect as adding an extra dimension to nature. Employing the Fourier theory, scientists began to observe nature in an additional dimension, i.e., the Fourier space, which brought a wonderful new source of intuition. This intuition led to numerous groundbreaking discoveries and tools[29-60] that have helped achieve our current level of technology and high standard of living. While Fourier may not be the greatest mathematician in history, he clearly is one of the most influential mathematicians in the history of science and technology.

Fourier analysis is an essential tool, widely used today in almost all areas of the physical and biological sciences.[29-82] References 29 to 56 all rely on Fourier analysis and were chosen as illustrations from dozens of published work that received more than 500 citations since 1965. To give the reader an idea of Fourier's impact, the total number of peer-reviewed works that use Fourier analysis constitutes ~0.5 % of *all the papers* published since 1970, *including* the social science papers. This high percentage is a clear indication of how vital the Fourier transform theory is to the advancement of science and technology. Important fields that depend heavily on Fourier transform analysis include: nuclear magnetic resonance and tomography,[31,35,43,44,48], acoustic imaging,[57,59] molecular imaging,[32,36,41,45,80] interferometry,[38,42,49] telescopic imaging,[34,50] astronomy and astrophysics,[50,51] X-ray diffraction,[45,53] spectroscopy,[47,48,54,62-79], quantum mechanics,[37,40] elipsometry,[55] digital image processing,[30,56,60], Fourier optics,[58] etc.

Following the development of computers, another significant milestone in the history of harmonic analysis was the invention of a fast Fourier transform algorithm[29] (known as FFT), which joined the power of computers to the power of Fourier analysis. All of the above-mentioned great technologies that rely on Fourier analysis are based on the FFT routine run by computers. The FFT algorithm can be considered as one of the most indispensable algorithms in science and technology since the invention of computers. The fact that the original paper of FFT [29] received ~3000 citations so far is a good indication of this.

The main focus of this dissertation is non-destructive characterization tools utilizing Fourier transform-based techniques. The key step for all these characterization tools is the recovery of the Fourier transform phase from the Fourier transform magnitude information *only*. The next section presents a brief introduction to the concept of phase and magnitude in Fourier transform theory.

1.2 FOURIER TRANSFORM PHASE AND MAGNITUDE

The one-dimensional Fourier transform (FT) of a function $g(t)$, where t represents any real variable, is defined as:

$$G(f) = \int_{-\infty}^{\infty} g(t) \cdot exp(-j \cdot 2\pi \cdot f \cdot t) \cdot dt \quad (1)$$

where f is the frequency variable in the Fourier domain, or Fourier space. The inverse Fourier transform is defined as:

$$g(t) = \int_{-\infty}^{\infty} G(f) \cdot exp(j \cdot 2\pi \cdot f \cdot t) \cdot df \quad (2)$$

In general, a complex $g(t)$ yields a complex $G(f)$. In the Fourier domain representation, for any given $g(t)$, one gets two different real functions: (1) the FT magnitude, $|G(f)|$; and (2) the FT phase, $\phi(f)$, where $G(f) = |G(f)| \cdot exp(j \cdot \phi(f))$. However, for certain special functions, a complex $g(t)$ can yield a real $G(f)$ or, a complex $G(f)$ can yield (in the inverse Fourier domain) a real $g(t)$. Essentially, the FT and inverse FT operations are duals of each other and do not cause any redundancy or any loss of information.

Physically, the FT magnitude at a particular frequency represents the strength or power of each frequency component that makes up the function $g(t)$. The square of the FT magnitude is often referred as the "power spectrum" of the function. Two functions that are totally different in the inverse Fourier domain can have the same power spectrum. The critical components that determine the behavior of the function in the inverse Fourier domain are the relative phases of all the Fourier amplitudes. If the phases of all the Fourier components are *locked*, i.e., the phase difference between any two adjacent Fourier components is constant all across the spectrum, then the function $g(t)$, which is often misleadingly referred as "transform limited", will have the smallest width in the inverse Fourier domain. Any additional relative phase difference between the adjacent Fourier components of the function simply broadens $g(t)$. In the limiting case, where the phases of the Fourier components vary randomly, $g(t)$ will have a noise-like behavior for any power spectrum (the exception being extremely narrow-band signals, such as a single-frequency function).

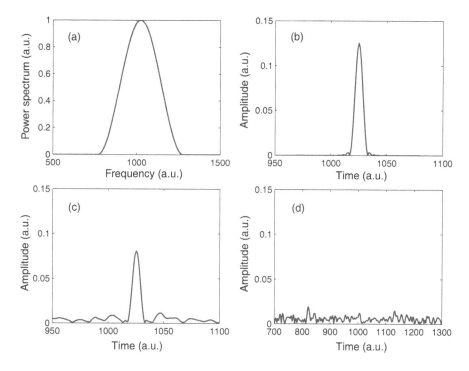

Fig. 2. (a) Arbitrarily assumed power spectrum; (b) phase locked signal amplitude corresponding to the power spectrum in (a); (c) signal amplitude when a uniform random FT phase (between $-\pi/2$ and $\pi/2$) is applied to the power spectrum in (a); (d) signal amplitude when a uniform random FT phase (between $-\pi$ and π) is applied to the power spectrum in (a).

The concept discussed above is illustrated in Fig. 2, where all the signal amplitudes shown in Figs. 2(b)-(d) have the same power spectrum, shown in Fig. 2(a). The only difference between these three time signals is their FT phase: in (b), a phase-locked case is illustrated; in (c), a uniform random phase that was allowed to vary between $-\pi/2$ and $\pi/2$ is illustrated; and in (d), a uniform random phase that was allowed to vary between $-\pi$ and π is shown. As previously discussed, the addition of the random phase broadens the time signal, and if the random phase is strong enough, it eventually yields a noise-like structure, as in Fig. 2(d). The FT phase clearly has an extremely important effect on the functional form of $g(t)$.

In the physical sciences, the measured quantities are often the FT magnitudes of the function of interest. For instance, in optics, the power spectrum of optical pulses is measured using a spectrum analyzer, which first disperses the input optical pulse into its frequency components using for example a grating, then records the power in each frequency component using a detector such as a charge coupled device. This power spectrum measurement requires a relatively simple instrument. Unfortunately, the FT phase measurements are not nearly as simple; direct phase measurements almost always require rather complex interferometric set-ups. Yet, in many physical problems the FT phase is absolutely essential in order to invert the whole complex FT to retrieve the original function using Eq. (2). Therefore in various fields involving a measurement of the FT of some physical parameter, there is a significant need for simpler techniques that can measure either directly or indirectly the FT phase.

1.3 CONTRIBUTION OF THIS WORK

The main theme of this thesis is the development of various nondestructive characterization tools based on FT theories. Because Fourier transform based techniques are widely used in most areas of science and technology, we were able to make significant contributions to several fields. Important contributions of this thesis include:

(1) Development of the analytical theory of FT spectral interferometry for nondestructive characterization of nonlinear thin films and its experimental demonstration.[5,9,10,12]

    a. Two-sample technique[10]

    b. Twin-sample technique[12]

    c. Reference-sample technique[9]

(2) Development of a powerful minimum phase function based iterative *non-interferometric* characterization tool, and its experimental demonstration for:

    a. Nonlinear thin film characterization[8]

       b.   Fiber Bragg grating characterization[1,7]

(3) First derivation of the full theoretical relationship between the classical Maker fringe curve and the FT of the measured nonlinearity profile.[5,12]

(4) Development of a cylinder-assisted Maker fringe technique to probe second-order nonlinear materials, and its experimental demonstration with a record high internal propagation angle approaching 90°.[11]

(5) First demonstration of the unambiguous recovery of the nonlinearity profile of thermally poled silica samples.[12]

(6) Demonstration of the highest reported peak nonlinear coefficient (~1.6 pm/V) in thermally poled germanosilicate glasses.[6]

(7) Development of a powerful technique for spectral interferometry based on minimum phase functions, which we call SIMBA.[4]

(8) Applications of SIMBA to:

       a.   uniquely characterize ultrashort optical pulses[4]

       b.   uniquely characterize fiber Bragg gratings[2]

       c.   improve the performance of existing frequency domain optical coherence tomography systems.[3]

(9) Design, fabrication and testing of poled germanium doped glass planar electro-optic modulators with the highest reported effective nonlinearity in poled integrated devices.

It should be emphasized that except for contributions (4), (6) and (9), which constitute important differential improvements over the previous results published in relevant literature, the development and demonstration of all other contributions constitutes a *breakthrough* when compared with the level of the prior art. The impact of these contributions will be further explored in the following chapters. The contributions listed above resulted in nine journal and twelve conference publications, all of which were peer-reviewed, and eight patent applications.[1-24]

1.4 ORGANIZATION OF THE DISSERTATION

Chapter 2 serves as a brief introduction to various FT phase recovery techniques developed in this thesis. Specifically, the concept of minimum phase functions is introduced, and its relationship to FT phase recovery is discussed. Furthermore, the basics of analytical spectral interferometry techniques for the same purpose of FT phase recovery are introduced.

Chapter 3 describes the characterization of second-order nonlinear materials, using analytical and iterative techniques based on Maker fringe measurements. Each technique is also demonstrated experimentally using thermally poled fused silica samples. The first part of Chapter 3 is a basic introduction to classical spectral interferometry techniques, whereas the second part is an introduction to the fundamental theory of minimum phase function based non-interferometric recovery techniques.

Chapter 4 reports the results of optimization of the induced nonlinearity profile in thermally poled germanosilicate glasses deposited on fused-silica substrates by plasma-enhanced chemical vapor deposition. Specifically, the recovered nonlinearity profiles of several different poled germanosilicate glass samples are presented, along with a discussion on the origin of the observed differences and similarities between the samples.

Chapter 5 explains the basics of SIMBA, as applied to recover the complex temporal profile of ultrashort pulses. The strengths and advantages of this technique over the existing tools are demonstrated using numerical simulations and experimental results.

Chapter 6 explores a non-interferometric technique based on minimum phase functions to uniquely relate the group delay and magnitude spectra of transmission fiber Bragg gratings (FBGs). This technique is discussed using both numerical simulations and experimental results.

Chapter 7 applies the core of the interferometric SIMBA technique developed in Chapter 5 to uniquely characterize FBGs. Its advantages over all existing techniques, including the non-interferometric approach presented in Chapter 6 are also reviewed.

Chapter 8 describes the advances that are possible by applying SIMBA to the field of optical coherence tomography (OCT), and numerically demonstrates its advantages for frequency domain OCT systems.

Chapter 9 briefly discusses two additional applications, where MPF concepts introduced in the early chapters can make a significant impact. The first part of the chapter describes the application of MPFs to optical image processing, while the second part of the chapter discusses the concept of SIMBA-based femtosecond spectroscopy.

Chapter 10 concludes with a brief summary of the key achievements of the dissertation, and briefly discusses future work.

REFERENCES

1. A. Ozcan, M. J. F. Digonnet, and G. S. Kino, "Iterative characterization and design of fiber Bragg gratings," *in preparation, to be submitted to Optics Express* (2005)

2. A. Ozcan, M. J. F. Digonnet, and G. S. Kino, "SIMBA technique to fully characterize fiber Bragg gratings," *in preparation, to be submitted to IEEE JQE* (2005)

3. A. Ozcan, M. J. F. Digonnet, and G. S. Kino, "Improvements in optical coherence tomography systems using minimum phase functions," *in preparation, to be submitted to Optics Express* (2005)

4. A. Ozcan, M. J. F. Digonnet, and G. S. Kino, "SIMBA technique to retrieve the phase and magnitude of the temporal profile of weak ultra-short laser pulses," Optics Express, *submitted* (2005)

5. A. Ozcan, M. J. F. Digonnet, G. S. Kino, "Detailed analysis of inverse Fourier transform techniques to uniquely infer second-order nonlinearity profile of thin films," J. Appl. Phys. 97, 013502 1, (2005)

6. A. Ozcan, M. J. F. Digonnet, G. S. Kino, F. Ay, and A. Aydinli, "Characterization of thermally poled germanosilicate thin films" Optics Express 12, 4698 (2004)

7. A. Ozcan, M. J. F. Digonnet, and G. S. Kino, "Group delay recovery using iterative processing of amplitude of transmission spectra of fibre Bragg gratings," Electron. Lett. 40, 1104 (2004)

8. A. Ozcan, M. J. F. Digonnet, and G. S. Kino, "Iterative processing of second-order optical nonlinearity depth profiles," Optics Express 12, 3367 (2004)

9. A. Ozcan, M. J. F. Digonnet, and G. S. Kino, "Simplified inverse Fourier transform technique to measure optical nonlinearity profiles using reference sample," Electron. Lett. 40, 551 (2004)

10. A. Ozcan, M. J. F. Digonnet, and G. S. Kino, "Improved technique to determine second-order optical nonlinearity profiles using two different samples," Appl. Phys. Lett. 84, 681 (2004)

11. A. Ozcan, M. J. F. Digonnet, and G. S. Kino, "Cylinder-assisted Maker fringe technique," Electron. Lett. 39, 1834 (2003)

12. A. Ozcan, M. J. F. Digonnet, and G. S. Kino, "Inverse Fourier Transform technique to determine second-order optical nonlinearity spatial profiles," Appl. Phys. Lett. 82, 1362 (2003)

13. A. Ozcan, M. J. F. Digonnet, G. S. Kino, "SIMBA: A new technique for ultrashort pulse characterization," *accepted to* IEEE LEOS Summer Topicals, 25-27 July 2005, San Diego, CA

14. A. Ozcan, M. J. F. Digonnet, G. S. Kino, F. Ay, and A. Aydinli, "Thermally poled germanosilicate films with high second-order nonlinearity," Conference on Lasers and Electro-optics (CLEO'05), 23-27 May 2005, Baltimore, MD

15. A. Ozcan, M. J. F. Digonnet, G. S. Kino, "Iterative characterization of the group delay properties of fiber Bragg gratings," Conference on Lasers and Electro-optics (CLEO'05), 23-27 May 2005, Baltimore, MD

16. A. Ozcan, M. J. F. Digonnet, G. S. Kino, "Dependence of the induced second-order optical nonlinearity profile of poled silica samples on poling conditions," SPIE Photonics West, 24-29 January 2005, San Jose, CA, paper # 5723-28

17. A. Ozcan, M. J. F. Digonnet, G. S. Kino, "Ultra-short laser pulse characterization using a reference laser pulse," SPIE Photonics West, 24-29 January 2005, San Jose, CA, paper # 5708-12

18. A. Ozcan, M. J. F. Digonnet, and G. S. Kino, "A simple post-processing technique to improve the retrieval accuracy of second-order nonlinearity profiles," in Proceedings of Conference on Lasers and Electro-optics (CLEO'04), OSA Technical Digest (Optical Society of America, Washington DC, 2004), paper CThJ6.

19. A. Ozcan, M. J. F. Digonnet, and G. S. Kino, "Comparison of three inverse Fourier transform techniques to determine the second-order optical nonlinearity profile of thin films," Proceedings of the SPIE - The International Society for Optical Engineering; 5451, 304 (2004)

20. A. Ozcan, M. J. F. Digonnet, and G. S. Kino, "Simplified inverse Fourier transform technique to determine second-order optical nonlinearity profiles using a reference sample," in Proceedings of Optical Fiber Communication Conference (OFC'04), OSA Technical Digest (Optical Society of America, Washington DC, 2004), paper FC3.

21. A. Ozcan, M. J. F. Digonnet, and G. S. Kino, "Cylinder-assisted Maker-fringe technique to probe second-order nonlinearity profiles," Proceedings of the SPIE - The International Society for Optical Engineering; 5350, 109 (2004)

22. A. Ozcan, M. J. F. Digonnet, and G. S. Kino, "Improved Fourier transform technique to determine second-order optical nonlinearity profiles," in Proceedings of Bragg Gratings, Photosensitivity and Poling in Glass Waveguides (BGPP'03), OSA Technical Digest (Optical Society of America, Washington DC, 2003), paper WB3.

23. A. Ozcan, M. J. F. Digonnet, and G. S. Kino, "A novel technique to determine second-order optical nonlinearity profiles," in Proceedings of Optical Fiber Communication Conference (OFC'03), OSA Technical Digest (Optical Society of America, Washington DC, 2003), paper ThM4.

24. U. L. Block, A. Ozcan, M. J. F. Digonnet, and M. M. Fejer, "Polarization-independent mechanically induced long-period fiber gratings," Proceedings of the SPIE - The International Society for Optical Engineering; 4638, 72 (2002)

25. Y. Katznelson, in *An introduction to Harmonic Analysis*, (Dover Publications, New York, 1976)

26. J. Herivel, *Joseph Fourier: The Man and the Physicist* (Oxford, 1975)

27. E. T. Bell, *Men of Mathematics*, (Touchstone Book, 1986)

28. http://fclass.vaniercollege.qc.ca/web/mathematics/about/history.htm

29. J. W. Tukey, and J. W. Cooley, "An algorithm for machine calculation of complex Fourier series," Mathematics of Computation 19, 297 (1965)

30. S. G. Mallat, "Theory for multiresolution signal decomposition: the wavelet representation," IEEE Transactions on Pattern Analysis and Machine Intelligence 11, 674 (1989)

31. F. Delaglio, *et al.*, "NMRPipe: A multidimensional spectral processing system based on UNIX pipes," Journal of Biomolecular NMR 6, 277 (1995)

32. T. A. Jones, "A graphics model building and refinement system for macromolecules," Journal of Applied Crystallography 11, 268 (1978)

33. J. D. Weeks, D. Chandler, and H. C. Andersen, "Role of repulsion forces in determining the equilibrium structure of simple liquids," Journal of Chemical Physics 12, 5237 (1971)

34. R. J. Read, "Improved Fourier coefficients for maps using phase from partial structures with errors," Acta Crystallographica Section A 42, 140 (1986)

35. A. Bax, and R. Freeman, "Investigation of complex networks of spin-spin coupling by two-dimensional NMR," Journal of Magnetic Resonance 44, 542 (1981)

36. A. Altomare, *et al.*, "SIR97: a new tool for crystal structure determination and refinement," Journal of Applied Crystallography 32, 115 (1999)

37. M. D. Feit, J. A. Fleck, and A. Steiger, "Solution of the Schrodinger equation by a spectral method," Journal of Computational Physics 47, 412 (1982)

38. F. W. Campbell, and J. G. Robson, "Application of Fourier analysis to visibility of gratings," Journal of Physiology 197, 551 (1968)

39. P. A. Stadelmann, "EMS- A software package for electron diffraction analysis and HREM image simulation in materials science," Ultramicroscopy 21, 131 (1987)

40. R. Kosloff, "Time-dependent quantum-mechanical methods for molecular dynamics," Journal of Physical Chemistry 92, 2087 (1988)

41. C. C. F. Blake, *et al.*, "Structure of hen egg-white lysozyme- a 3-dimensional Fourier synthesis at 2A resolution," Nature 206, 757 (1965)

42. J. A. Hogbom, "Aperture synthesis with a non-regular distribution of interferometer baselines," Astronomy and Astrophysics Supplement 15, 417 (1974)

43. P. A. Bandettini, A. Jesmanowicz, A. Wong, and E. C. Hyde, "Processing strategies for time-course data sets in functional MRI of the human brain," Magnetic Resonance in Medicine 30, 161 (1993)

44. P. J. Hore, "Solvent suppression in Fourier transform nuclear magnetic resonance," Journal of Magnetic Resonance 55, 283 (1983)

45. D. E. Sayers, E. A. Stern, and F. W. Lytle, "New technique for investigating noncrystalline structures: Fourier analysis of the extended X-ray absorption fine structure," Phys. Rev. Lett. 27, 1204 (1971)

46. J. K. Kauppinen, *et al.*, "Fourier self-deconvolution: a method for resolving intrinsically overlapped bands," Applied Spectroscopy 35, 271 (1981)

47. T. J. Balle, and W. H. Flygare, "Fabry-Perot cavity pulsed Fourier transform microwave spectrometer with a pulsed nozzle particle source," Review of Scientific Instruments 52, 33 (1981)

48. R. R. Ernest, and W. A Anderson, "Application of Fourier transform spectroscopy to magnetic resonance," Review of Scientific Instruments 37, 93 (1966)

49. M. Takeda, H. Ina, and S. Kobayashi, "Fourier transform method of fringe pattern analysis for computer based topography and interferometry," J. Opt. Soc. Am. 72, 156 (1982)

50. S. M. Faber, and R. E. Jackson, "Velocity dispersion and mass-to-light ratios for elliptical galaxies," Astrophysical Journal 204, 668 (1976)

51. A. Labeyrie, "Attainment of diffraction limited resolution in large telescopes by Fourier analyzing speckle patterns in star images," Astronomy and Astrophysics 6, 85 (1970)

52. G. B. Benedek, "Theory of transparency of the eye," Applied Optics 10, 459 (1971)

53. M. F. Perutz, *et al.*, "Structure of haemoglobin - 3-dimensional Fourier synthesis at 5.5 A resolution obtained by X-ray analysis," Nature 185, 416 (1960)

54. W. K. Surewicz, H. H. Mantsch, and D. Chapman, "Determination of the protein secondary structure by Fourier transform infrared spectroscopy: A critical assessment," Biochemistry 32, 389 (1993)

55. D. E. Aspnes, and A. A. Studna, "High precision scanning elipsometer," Applied Optics 14, 220 (1975)

56. D. Mendlovic, and H. M. Ozaktas, "Fractional Fourier transforms and their optical implementation – I," J. Opt. Soc. Am. A 10, 1875 (1993)

57. R. K. Mueller, M. Kaveh, and G. Vade, "Reconstructive tomography and applications to ultrasonics," Proceedings of the IEEE 67, 567 (1979)

58. J. W. Goodman, *Introduction to Fourier Optics*, (Mc Graw-Hill, New York, 2002)

59. G. S. Kino, *Acoustic Waves: Devices, Imaging, and Analog Signal Processing*, (Prentice Hall, New Jersey, 1987)

60. K. R. Castleman, in *Digital Image Processing*, (Prentice Hall, New Jersey, 1979)

61. V. Oppenheim, and R. W. Schafer, *Digital Signal Processing*, (Prentice Hall, 2002), Chap. 7.

62. F. Reynaud, F. Salin, and A. Barthelemy, "Measurement of phase shifts introduced by nonlinear optical phenomena on subpicosecond pulses," Opt. Lett. 14, 275 (1989)

63. E. Tokunaga, A. Terasaki, and T. Kobayashi, "Frequency-domain interferometer for femtosecond time-resolved phase spectroscopy," Opt. Lett. 17, 1131 (1992)

64. E. Tokunaga, A. Terasaki, and T. Kobayashi, "Induced phase modulation of chirped continuum pulses studied with a femtosecond frequency-domain interferometer," Opt. Lett. 18, 370 (1993)

65. J. P. Geindre *et al.*, "Frequency-domain interferometer for measuring the phase and amplitude of a femtosecond pulse probing a laser-produced plasma," Opt. Lett. 19, 1997 (1994)

66. C. W. Siders *et al.*, "Laser wakefield excitation and measurement by femtosecond longitudinal interferometry," Phys. Rev. Lett. 76, 3570 (1996)

67. L. Lepetit, G. Cheriaux, and M. Joffre, "Linear techniques of phase measurement by femtosecond spectral interferometry for applications in spectroscopy," J. Opt. Soc. Am. B 12, 2467 (1995)

68. S. M. Ghallager, *et al.*, "Heterodyne detection of the complete electric field of femtosecond four-wave mixing signals," J. Opt. Soc. Am. B 15, 2338 (1998)

69. J. Tignon, M. V. Marquezini, T. Hasche, and D. S. Chemla, "Spectral interferometry of semiconductor nanostructures," IEEE J. Quantum Electron. 35, 510 (1999)

70. X. Chen, *et al.*, "Temporally and spectrally resolved amplitude and phase of coherent four-wave-mixing emission from GaAs quantum wells," Phys. Rev. B 56, 9738 (1997)

71. D. Birkedal, and J. Shah, "Femtosecond spectral interferometry of resonant secondary emission from quantum wells: Resonance Rayleigh scattering in the nonergodic regime," Phys. Rev. Lett. 81, 2372 (1998)

72. A. F. Fercher, C. K. Hitzenberger, G. Kamp, and S. Y. El-Zaiat, "Measurement of intraocular distances by backscattering spectral interferometry," Opt. Commun. **117**, 43-48 (1995)

73. G. Hausler and M. W. Lindler, "Coherence radar and spectral radar- New tools for dermatological diagnosis," J. Biomed. Opt. **3**, 21-31 (1998)

74. M. Wojtkowski, R. A. Leitgeb, A. Kowalczyk, T. Bajraszewski, and A. F. Fercher, "In vivo human retinal imaging by Fourier domain optical coherence tomography", J. Biomed. Opt. **7**, 457-463, (2003)

75. D. N. Fittinghoff, *et al.*, "Measurement of the intensity and phase of ultraweak, ultrashort laser pulses", Opt. Lett. 21, 884 (1996)

76. C. Iaconis and I. A. Walmsley, "Spectral phase interferometry for direct electric-field reconstruction of ultrashort optical pulses", Opt. Lett. 23, 792 (1998)

77. S. Keren and M. Horowitz, "Interrogation of fiber gratings by use of low-coherence spectral interferometry of noiselike pulses," Opt. Lett. **26**, 328 (2001)

78. C. Dorrer, N. Belabas, J.P. Likforman, and M. Joffre, "Spectral resolution and sampling issues in Fourier-transform spectral interferometry," J. Opt. Soc. Am. B 17, 1795 (2000)

79. C. Dorrer, "Influence of the calibration of the detector on spectral interferometry," J. Opt. Soc. Am. B 16, 1160 (1999)

80. J. M. Zuo, *et al.*, "Atomic resolution imaging of a carbon nanotube from diffraction intensities," Science 300, 1419 (2003)

81. J. R. Fienup, "Reconstruction of an object from the modulus of its Fourier transform," Opt. Lett. 3, 27 (1978).

82. R. W. Gerchberg and W. O. Saxton, "Practical algorithm for the determination of phase from image and diffraction plane pictures," Optik **35**, 237-246 (1972)

CHAPTER 2: INTRODUCTION TO FOURIER TRANSFORM PHASE RECOVERY USING SPECTRAL INTERFEROMETRY AND MINIMUM PHASE FUNCTIONS

If I have a thousand ideas and only one turns out to be good, I am satisfied.
Alfred Nobel

This chapter aims to give a brief introduction to the machinery used in this thesis to recover vital information about various physical phenomena.[1-6] All the problems discussed in this thesis involve a measurement of the Fourier transform (FT) magnitude of the physical function of interest, such as the second-order optical nonlinearity depth profile of thin films, the complex electric-field profile of ultrashort laser pulses, the reflection impulse response of fiber Bragg gratings (FBGs) or the field scattering function of tissue samples. In order to recover the physical function we need the FT phase as well. The recovery of the missing FT phase is achieved using various tools, specifically designed for the field of interest. Starting next section, we introduce the underlying principles of these tools.

2.1 FOURIER TRANSFORM PHASE RECOVERY FROM FOURIER TRANSFORM MAGNITUDE

This dissertation discusses various approaches for the recovery of the FT phase from FT magnitude measurements only. These approaches can be divided into two categories: (1) analytical techniques, and (2) iterative techniques. Analytical techniques rely on spectral interferometry and can uniquely recover the FT phase from FT magnitude measurements. However, they require either the generation of mirror images of functions (e.g., generation of $f(-t)$ from $f(t)$) or the *priori* knowledge of a reference function. These requirements are not easy to satisfy in many fields. On the other hand, iterative approaches rely on the properties of a special family of functions called minimum-phase functions (MPFs) and are applicable to fields where the function of interest is naturally or can be artificially made either an exact MPF or close to one. As we will show, this case is far more prevalent, and iterative techniques can be applied to a large number of fields in physics and chemistry. In this thesis, different fields that significantly benefit from these analytical and iterative approaches are discussed.

2.1.1 ANALYTICAL PHASE RECOVERY

Spectral interferometry[7-24] forms the basis of the analytical phase recovery techniques discussed in this thesis. In the past, spectral interferometry (SI) has been applied to problems in several fields, including but not limited to Fourier transform femtosecond spectroscopy,[7-16] frequency domain optical coherence tomography,[17-19] ultrashort pulse characterization,[20-21] and fiber Bragg grating characterization.[22]

In general, the principle of SI relies on recording the power spectrum generated as a result of the interference between two functions, one serving as the reference function and the other as the sample function to be characterized. Because of the interference between the various frequency components of the two functions, the difference in FT phase between the two functions becomes part of the measured power spectrum. The classical approach in modern spectral interferometry uses an analytical inverse FT (IFT) processing technique [12,23,24] to recover this phase difference from the recorded power spectrum. For applications such as femtosecond spectroscopy,[7-16] the recovered FT phase difference may be adequate; for other applications, such as ultrashort pulse characterization, additional information is needed, for example the FT phase of the reference function.[20]

In the first half of Chapter 3, the above-described *analytical IFT* approach of SI is applied to characterize the depth profile of nonlinear thin films. In light of the relevant work published prior to our work, as discussed in Chapter 3, the breakthrough of our approach for *nonlinear optics* is unquestionable. Our contributions enabled us to characterize uniquely the second-order optical nonlinear profile of thin films that was not possible before these techniques were developed. This is especially important to optimize the design and fabrication of electro-optic devices such as modulators or switches. More importantly, compared to all previous SI-related applications, the analytical IFT techniques[25-27] discussed in Chapter 3 are unique: they involve artificially creating mirror images of physical functions, such that creating $g(-t)$ from $g(t)$, by simply rotating the nonlinear sample by 180°. In other fields, such as femtosecond spectroscopy, ultrashort pulse characterization and FBG characterization, the equivalent operation of creating a mirror image of the function of interest requires *full electric field time reversal* of ultrashort pulses, which is quite difficult to achieve, if not impossible, especially for sub-picosecond pulses. In nonlinear optics, the possibility of artificially creating the mirror image of a nonlinearity profile by simply rotating the sample by 180° enabled us to invent unique SI techniques, such as the two-sample technique[26] described in Chapter 3.

2.1.2 ITERATIVE PHASE RECOVERY

All the iterative phase recovery techniques discussed in this thesis are based on MPFs. Before we introduce the details of the phase recovery process, it is important to gain a sound understanding of MPFs. The next section aims to provide this essential understanding.

2.1.2.1 Basic properties of minimum phase functions

In general, the FT phase of a one-dimensional function cannot be recovered from only the FT magnitude of this function. One exception is MPFs, a special family of functions that have the unique property that their FT phase and magnitude are related through an analytical relationship, i.e., the Hilbert transform.[1]

The first defining property of MPFs is that all MPFs are causal.[1] This condition is almost always satisfied for physical functions. However, it does not mean that all causal functions have to be MPFs. In terms of its mathematical definition, an MPF is characterized by having a z-transform with all its poles and zeros on or inside the unit circle.[1] If this condition is satisfied, the function is by definition causal and more importantly not an ordinary causal function *but an MPF*. In other words, a function is an MPF *if and only if* all the poles and zeros of its z-transform lie on or inside the unit circle.

The z-transform for a sequence $x(n)$ is defined as $X(z) = \sum_{n=-\infty}^{\infty} x(n) \cdot z^{-n}$, where n is an integer that numbers sampled values of the function variable, and z represents the complex variable of the z-transform and should *not* be confused with the space variable in nonlinear thin films.[1] This pole-zero constraint can be considered to be an easy metric to test whether or not a causal function is an MPF, since the numerical computation of a z-transform is quite simple and fast using a computer.

As rigorous as it is, this mathematical definition fails to provide a physical picture of what an MPF looks like. To better understand intuitively which physical functions are likely to be an MPF, let us denote an MPF by $d_{min}(n)$. Note the function $d_{min}(n)$ can be a real or a complex quantity. First, all MPFs must be causal, where causality condition is mathematically *defined* as $d_{min}(n)=0$ for $n < 0$. However, any function that has a finite extent (a condition that almost all physical functions satisfy) can be transformed into a causal function by a shift of origin. Second, the energy of a minimum-phase function, which is defined as $\sum_{n=0}^{m-1} |\, d_{min}(n)\,|^2$ for m samples of the function $d_{min}(n)$, must satisfy the inequality [1]

$$\sum_{n=0}^{m-1}|d_{min}(n)|^2 \geq \sum_{n=0}^{m-1}|d(n)|^2 \qquad (1)$$

for all possible values of $m > 0$. In Eq. (1), $d(n)$ represents any of the infinite number of functions that have the same FT magnitude as $d_{min}(n)$. Another property worth mentioning is that:

$$|d_{min}(0)| \geq |d(0)| \qquad (2)$$

This last inequality can be derived from Eq. (1) by setting $m = 1$. These two properties of MPFs (Eqs. (1) and (2)) suggest that most of the energy of $d_{min}(n)$ is concentrated around $n = 0$.[1] Stated differently, *any causal function, complex or real, with a dominant peak close to the origin will be either a minimum-phase function or close to one.* To illustrate this point, we plotted in Fig. 1 several causal functions that have a dominant peak close to the origin, which makes them an exact MPF (except the rectangular function). For the rectangular function, which is not an exact MPF but is close to one, the intuition that an MPF has a dominant peak close to the origin can be still considered to be valid.

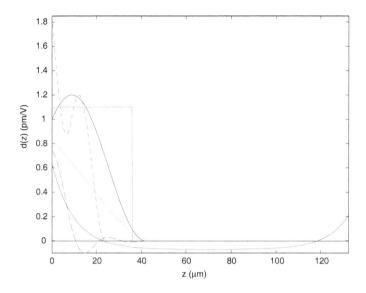

Fig. 1. Examples of causal functions that are either exact MPFs or close to being one, i.e., they can be recovered fully from their FT magnitudes.

Now that we have an intuitive understanding on which physical functions can be an MPF, the question is how to extract the FT phase information from only the FT magnitude for this family of special functions. The next section addresses this important question.

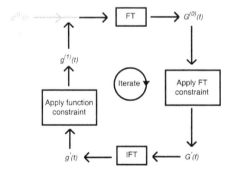

Fig. 2. General block diagram of the iterative error-reduction algorithm.

2.1.2.2 FT phase recovery for MPFs

As mentioned earlier, it is well known that for MPFs, the FT phase and magnitude are analytically related through the Hilbert transform.[1] However, because of some of the difficulties in the numerical evaluation of Hilbert transform (such as phase unwrapping and noise sensitivity[1-4]), in this dissertation we have used a different mechanism, generally known as iterative-error-reduction algorithm such as Fienup[5] or Gerchberg-Saxton algorithms[6], for extracting the FT phase information from the FT magnitude measurements. Iterative error-reduction algorithms are well-known computation tools that have been widely used in fields such as image processing, electron microscopy, astronomy, etc. In this family of algorithms, as outlined in Fig. 2, an initial estimate $g^{(0)}(t)$ of a function $g(t)$ is improved after each iteration, using the known constraints of the function and of its Fourier transform (FT) $G(f)$. These constraints can be any partial information that is known to be true, such as that the function is causal or has a known FT phase or magnitude spectrum. For a function that is known to be an MPF, in the most general case the constraint is that it is causal (or has finite extent). Depending on the physical problem, additional constraints can be applied, for example if the function is a real quantity or is limited in space or time.

Given an initial estimate $g^{(0)}(t)$ of a target function $g(t)$, the first step of the error-reduction algorithm (Fig. 2) is to take the FT of $g^{(0)}(t)$, which yields $G^{(0)}(f)$. Next, the known constraint in the Fourier domain is applied to $G^{(0)}(f)$, which is followed by computing the IFT of the new function. This step yields an intermediate function $g'(t)$. The final step of the first iteration loop is to apply the function constraint (Fig. 2) to $g'(t)$, which yields a first estimate $g^{(1)}(t)$ of the target function $g(t)$. At the end of the n-th iteration, the error of the estimated function $g^{(n)}(t)$, which is defined as $\int \left| g(t) - g^{(n)}(t) \right|^2 dt / \int \left| g(t) \right|^2 dt$, is reduced. As will be explored in greater detail in the following chapters, of the infinite number of functions whose FT magnitude is equal to the FT magnitude input in the iterative loop, the algorithm converges, using only the causality property of MPFs as the function constraint, to the one and only one which is a minimum-phase function. For all the functions that are shown in Fig. 1, the recovery of each function from *only* its FT magnitude using this iterative approach (Fig. 2) is extremely accurate, with an error less than 4 x 10^{-3}%. This accuracy level was achieved after only 100 iterations, which took only a few seconds on a 500-MHz computer.

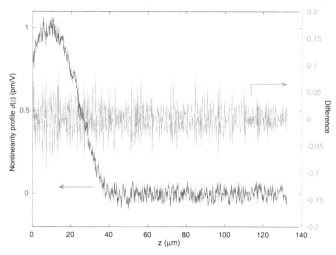

Fig. 3. The same buried-Gaussian profile as in Fig. 1 with uniform noise added. The result of the recovery with 100 iterations is also shown. The difference between the original noisy function and the recovered function is plotted on the left scale.

To explore the robustness and usefulness of this algorithm, we evaluated its accuracy for a number of functions other than minimum-phase functions. In a first series of simulations, uniform random noise (~14% peak-to-peak) was added to the profiles of Fig. 1, which were thus no longer MPFs. Because of the added random noise, most of the zeros of the noisy sequence's z-transform are no longer inside the unit circle. In all cases, the profiles recovered using the iterative loop of Fig. 2, after 100 iterations, from the FT magnitudes alone were in excellent agreement with the original noisy profile (average error under ~1.4%), as illustrated in Fig. 3 for an exemplary profile (buried Gaussian). The iterative error-reduction algorithm clearly works well, even in the presence of noise.

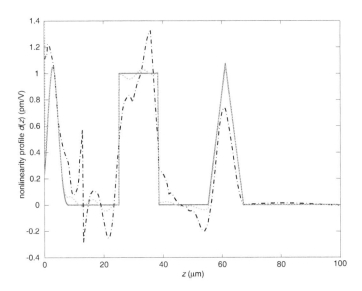

Fig. 4. An arbitrarily three-peaked function (solid curve) and the profile recovered (dot-dashed curve) with the iterative error-reduction algorithm after 100 iterations. The dotted curve shows the recovered profile when the magnitude of the function at the origin is increased by 10 times.

In a second series of simulations, we investigated profiles with several peaks of comparable magnitude. Because none of the peaks is dominant, such profiles do not satisfy Eqs. (1)-(2) and are not minimum-phase functions. We found that with two peaks of comparable magnitude, the algorithm's prediction is only marginally degraded and still quite acceptable. For example, when the peaks in the two-peak function of Fig. 1 are of comparable height, the recovered profile is still essentially indistinguishable from the original profile: the average error in the recovery increases to only 0.1%. With three peaks of comparable height (see Fig. 4), even though the iterative algorithm is not nearly as accurate as in the previous examples, the recovered profile still provides a decent estimate of the original profile. These simulations demonstrate that the iterative error-reduction algorithm (Fig. 2) is certainly not limited to minimum-phase functions.

2.2 CHARACTERIZATION TECHNIQUES BASED ON FOURIER TRANSFORM MAGNITUDE MEASUREMENTS

The analytical or iterative phase recovery techniques discussed in the previous section all require the measurement of an FT magnitude of a target function. In general, characterization techniques based on FT magnitude measurements can be grouped into two categories: (1) non-interferometric, and (2) interferometric. The basic distinction between these two categories is that for non-interferometric techniques the function of interest happens to be by definition (naturally) an MPF, which allows the FT phase to be recovered from a measurement of the FT magnitude spectrum *alone*. This recovery is achieved using the iterative phase recovery technique discussed in Section 2.1.2. On the other hand, interferometric characterization techniques are applied to fields where the function of interest is not an MPF, which makes the non-interferometric iterative approach fail.

2.2.1 NON-INTERFEROMETRIC CHARACTERIZATION TECHNIQUES

To be able to use non-interferometric characterization techniques, the function of interest must be an MPF or close to one. The missing FT phase can then be recovered from the measured FT magnitude of the function of interest *alone* by using the MPF-based iterative error-reduction algorithm of Fig. 2. This provides an exciting opportunity since a vital piece of information (the FT phase) can now be recovered from only a simple non-interferometric FT magnitude measurement of the function of interest.

In this thesis, two important fields that by definition have MPFs are discussed as examples of *non-interferometric* FT phase recovery from FT magnitude. Specifically, this characterization technique is used to uniquely recover the nonlinearity profile of thin films in the second half of Chapter 3 and in Chapter 4, and to uniquely characterize FBGs in Chapter 6.

2.2.2 INTERFEROMETRIC CHARACTERIZATION TECHNIQUES

As stated above, the exciting opportunity of the *non-interferometric* characterization tools of the previous section is limited to fields where the function of interest happens to be an MPF or close to one. However, in many fields this is not the case, and for these fields interferometric characterization techniques can be used.

There are two different approaches to interferometric characterization techniques. The first approach relies on analytical phase recovery using the classical spectral interferometry (Section 2.1.1). It is applicable to fields where either an already known reference function or a mirror image of the function of interest is available. As will be discussed in Chapter 3, these conditions are relatively easy to satisfy for nonlinear thin films, which made this approach a perfect tool to map the nonlinearity profile of thin films.

However, in general the above requirements of the classical spectral interferometry are challenging to meet for many fields. The second interferometric characterization technique, which relies on iterative phase recovery (Section 2.1.2), offers a solution to such fields. In this second approach, by a special arrangement in the experimental system, the measured function is *artificially* transformed into a new function that is to close to an MPF. As we illustrate further on, one of the main contributions of this thesis is to realize that even if a function is far from being an MPF, it is possible to turn it into either an exact MPF or into a function that is close to an MPF by simply adding a sharp dominant peak close to the origin (see Fig. 5). The effect of this added dominant peak is *to transform the whole composite function, complex or real, into an exact MPF or in some other cases into a function that is close to an MPF*. Once this is achieved, the FT magnitude spectrum of the composite function is measured and the composite function can be recovered using for instance the iterative error-reduction algorithm (Fig. 5).

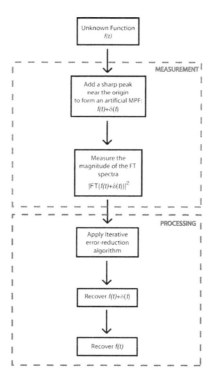

Fig. 5. General block diagram of artificially creating an MPF and its recovery.

The acronym of this general technique is *SIMBA*, which stands for spectral interferometry using minimum-phase based algorithms. The discovery of SIMBA historically originated from the quest to apply the success of MPF-based algorithms to other fields in particular the measurement of the temporal profile of an ultrashort pulse. As already discussed, for many fields, the function of interest does not satisfy the MPF constraints. For instance, in ultrafast optical pulse characterization, a typical pulse is generally far away from an MPF. Adding a sharp pulse to it, however, is a trivial matter, and this operation does turn it into an MPF or close to one. This sharp pulse can be provided by a different laser source or it can even be a tailored (e.g., compressed) version of the pulse to be characterized (refer to Chapter 5 for a detailed discussion). The same is also true for the scattering function of tissue samples, a parameter of interest for optical coherence tomography systems. As illustrated in Chapter 8, SIMBA can in this case be implemented by using a reference mirror, which acts as a Dirac-delta function. In Chapters 7 and 9, SIMBA is also applied to other problems, namely FBG characterization, optical image processing, and femtosecond spectroscopy.

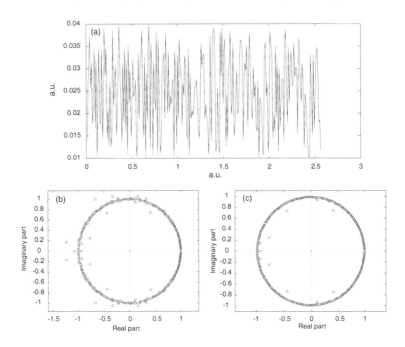

Fig. 6. (a) An arbitrarily chosen causal non-MPF, $f(t)$; (b) the pole-zero plot of the z-transform of $f(t)$; (c) the pole-zero plot of the z-transform of $\delta(t) + f(t)$.

To illustrate the effect of forming a composite function with a dominant peak at or close to the origin, we show in Fig. 6(a) an example of a non-MPF causal function, $f(t)$, arbitrarily chosen. Since many of the zeros of its z-transform are outside the unit circle (Fig. 6(b)), $f(t)$ is not an MPF. However, by adding to $f(t)$ another function that has a sharp peak at the origin, e.g., a Dirac-delta function, $\delta(t)$, we artificially construct an MPF. That this new function $\delta(t) + f(t)$ is an MPF is illustrated in the pole-zero plot of its z-transform (Fig. 6(c)). This figure shows that all the zeros of its z-transform are inside the unit circle. The recovery of the composite MPF, $\delta(t) + f(t)$, can now be *uniquely* achieved from only its FT magnitude information, using the iterative approach given in

Fig. 2. The same effect can also be achieved even if the added function is not a Dirac-delta function provided that it satisfies certain constraints that vary from field to field. A further discussion of this issue will be given in Chapters 5 and 7. To further illustrate this concept with another example, for the three-peaked function of Fig. 4, if the amplitude at the origin is increased by 10 times, the new recovered profile (dotted curve in Fig. 4) is significantly closer to the original profile.

2.3 CONCLUSIONS

In this chapter, the fundamentals of the tools used in this thesis to recover a function of interest from only its FT magnitude spectrum are discussed. The techniques used in this dissertation can be grouped into (1) analytical, and (2) iterative techniques. The analytical approach is based on classical spectral interferometry, and it allows the recovery of the FT phase uniquely using a simple analytical IFT based data processing. This technique is especially well suited for fields where generating mirror image of a function is easy to achieve, such as second-order optical nonlinearity depth profile of thin films.

The iterative techniques, on the other hand, are all based on MPFs and they require the use of an iterative error-reduction algorithm. This group of techniques is applicable to any function that is either an exact MPF or close to one. If the function of interest is naturally an MPF, then the technique is called *non-interferometric,* since all it requires the FT magnitude measurement of the function *alone.* However, when the function is not an MPF, which is generally the case, this simple approach fails. For such cases, adding to the function a sharp dominant peak at or close to its origin transforms the original function into either an exact MPF or close to one, which then makes it possible to apply an iterative error-reduction algorithm to the measured FT magnitude spectrum of this new function to uniquely recover the unknown function. This is the basic concept of the *interferometric* technique. This powerful technique is applicable to numerous fields of physics and chemistry, such as optical coherence tomography and femtosecond spectroscopy, as will be discussed in the following chapters.

REFERENCES

1. V. Oppenheim, and R. W. Schafer, *Digital Signal Processing*, (Prentice Hall, 2002), Chap. 7.

2. A. Ozcan, M. J. F. Digonnet, and G. S. Kino, "Group delay recovery using iterative processing of amplitude of transmission spectra of fibre Bragg gratings," Electron. Lett. 40, 1104 (2004)

3. T. F. Quatieri, Jr., and A. V. Oppenheim, "Iterative techniques for minimum phase signal reconstruction from phase or magnitude," IEEE Trans. Acoust., Speech, Signal Processing 29, 1187 (1981)

4. M. Hayes, J. S. Lim, and A. V. Oppenheim, "Signal reconstruction from phase or magnitude," IEEE Trans. Acoust., Speech, Signal Processing 28, 672 (1980)

5. J. R. Fienup, "Reconstruction of an object from the modulus of its Fourier transform," Opt. Lett. 3, 27 (1978).

6. R. W. Gerchberg and W. O. Saxton, "Practical algorithm for the determination of phase from image and diffraction plane pictures," Optik **35**, 237-246 (1972)

7. F. Reynaud, F. Salin, and A. Barthelemy, "Measurement of phase shifts introduced by nonlinear optical phenomena on subpicosecond pulses," Opt. Lett. 14, 275 (1989)

8. E. Tokunaga, A. Terasaki, and T. Kobayashi, "Frequency-domain interferometer for femtosecond time-resolved phase spectroscopy," Opt. Lett. 17, 1131 (1992)

9. E. Tokunaga, A. Terasaki, and T. Kobayashi, "Induced phase modulation of chirped continuum pulses studied with a femtosecond frequency-domain interferometer," Opt. Lett. 18, 370 (1993)

10. J. P. Geindre *et al.*, "Frequency-domain interferometer for measuring the phase and amplitude of a femtosecond pulse probing a laser-produced plasma," Opt. Lett. 19, 1997 (1994)

11. C. W. Siders *et al.*, "Laser wakefield excitation and measurement by femtosecond longitudinal interferometry," Phys. Rev. Lett. 76, 3570 (1996)

12. L. Lepetit, G. Cheriaux, and M. Joffre, "Linear techniques of phase measurement by femtosecond spectral interferometry for applications in spectroscopy," J. Opt. Soc. Am. B 12, 2467 (1995)

13. S. M. Ghallager, *et al.*, "Heterodyne detection of the complete electric field of femtosecond four-wave mixing signals," J. Opt. Soc. Am. B 15, 2338 (1998)

14. J. Tignon, M. V. Marquezini, T. Hasche, and D. S. Chemla, "Spectral interferometry of semiconductor nanostructures," IEEE J. Quantum Electron. 35, 510 (1999)

15. X. Chen, *et al.*, "Temporally and spectrally resolved amplitude and phase of coherent four-wave-mixing emission from GaAs quantum wells," Phys. Rev. B 56, 9738 (1997)

16. D. Birkedal, and J. Shah, "Femtosecond spectral interferometry of resonant secondary emission from quantum wells: Resonance Rayleigh scattering in the nonergodic regime," Phys. Rev. Lett. 81, 2372 (1998)

17. A. F. Fercher, C. K. Hitzenberger, G. Kamp, and S. Y. El-Zaiat, "Measurement of intraocular distances by backscattering spectral interferometry," Opt. Commun. **117**, 43-48 (1995)

18. G. Hausler and M. W. Lindler, "Coherence radar and spectral radar- New tools for dermatological diagnosis," J. Biomed. Opt. **3**, 21-31 (1998)

19. M. Wojtkowski, R. A. Leitgeb, A. Kowalczyk, T. Bajraszewski, and A. F. Fercher, "In vivo human retinal imaging by Fourier domain optical coherence tomography", J. Biomed. Opt. **7**, 457-463, (2003)

20. D. N. Fittinghoff, *et al.,* "Measurement of the intensity and phase of ultraweak, ultrashort laser pulses", Opt. Lett. 21, 884 (1996)

21. C. Iaconis and I. A. Walmsley, "Spectral phase interferometry for direct electric-field reconstruction of ultrashort optical pulses", Opt. Lett. 23, 792 (1998)

22. S. Keren and M. Horowitz, "Interrogation of fiber gratings by use of low-coherence spectral interferometry of noiselike pulses," Opt. Lett. **26**, 328 (2001)

23. C. Dorrer, N. Belabas, J.P. Likforman, and M. Joffre, "Spectral resolution and sampling issues in Fourier-transform spectral interferometry," J. Opt. Soc. Am. B 17, 1795 (2000)

24. C. Dorrer, "Influence of the calibration of the detector on spectral interferometry," J. Opt. Soc. Am. B 16, 1160 (1999)

25. A. Ozcan, M. J. F. Digonnet, G. S. Kino, "Inverse Fourier transform technique to determine second-order optical nonlinearity spatial profiles," Appl. Phys. Lett. 82, 1362 (2003)

26. A. Ozcan, M. J. F. Digonnet, G. S. Kino, "Improved technique to determine second-order optical nonlinearity profiles using two different samples," Appl. Phys. Lett. 84, 681 (2004)

27. A. Ozcan, M. J. F. Digonnet, and G. S. Kino, "Simplified inverse Fourier transform technique to measure optical nonlinearity profiles using reference sample," Electron. Lett. 40, 551 (2004)

CHAPTER 3: CHARACTERIZATION OF SECOND-ORDER OPTICAL NONLINEARITY DEPTH PROFILES

This chapter concerns the characterization of second-order optical nonlinearity depth profiles using spectral interferometry and minimum phase function (MPF) concepts. The first part of the chapter will discuss analytical tools that can uniquely recover the nonlinearity depth profile of second-order nonlinear crystals; the second part will discuss an iterative approach based on MPFs that can be used for the same purpose. Historically, the work given in this chapter enabled us to derive various characterization tools used for a wide range of physical problems. Initially, the analytical characterization tools based on spectral interferometry were developed to uniquely characterize second-order optical nonlinearity profile of thin films. Following this discovery, an iterative non-interferometric technique was developed to improve the accuracy of the analytical techniques by reducing the artificial "ringing" in the recovered profiles. Later, we discovered that the same iterative technique could actually be used to recover the nonlinearity profile of the thin film. This simple non-interferometric approach was then applied to various other fields to develop powerful non-destructive characterization techniques.

3.1 INTRODUCTION

Determining the second-order optical nonlinearity depth profile of various nonlinear thin films is an important yet challenging task. First, to control the fabrication process of various nonlinear thin films, an accurate tool to determine the nonlinearity profile of the thin film is needed. For some nonlinear materials such as poled glasses, which will be discussed in greater detail in Section 3.2.4.1, knowledge of this profile is essential to understand the physical origin of the nonlinearity, and it might also assist in developing methods to improve the strength, depth, and/or uniformity of the nonlinear region. Second, for fabrication of electro-optic devices, such as modulators or switches, the knowledge of the profile of the nonlinear region is crucial to optimize the design of the device by maximizing the overlap of the optical mode and the modulating electric-field with the nonlinear region. Therefore, we can conclude that for any field that deals with optical nonlinear thin films, characterization of the nonlinearity depth profile of the film is important. However, this task is quite challenging, as will be further explored in Section 3.2.1, especially for thin and weak nonlinear materials (with a total nonlinear region thickness of <50 μm and a peak nonlinear coefficient of <5 pm/V).

In the past, the most commonly used method to measure this nonlinearity profile was the Maker fringe (MF) technique.[7] However the classical MF measurement, as will be proved in Section 3.2.1, cannot provide a unique depth profile for a nonlinear thin film. In other words, one can easily come up with many different physically possible nonlinearity profiles given an MF measurement. A typical remedy is to assume that the profile has a certain shape (such as a top hat or a Gaussian) and to fit it to the MF data.[8-9] This approach of course does not yield reliable profile predictions. To circumvent this fundamental problem of the classical MF technique, some other approaches were proposed that involve etching of the nonlinear thin film, while the second-harmonic signal generated from the nonlinear region is still being detected.[10-11] These techniques are (1) destructive since they etch away the nonlinear material, and (2) still have problems of retrieving a unique solution to the nonlinearity depth profile, since in most cases the etching process dynamically changes the remaining part of the nonlinearity profile.

In the sections to follow, this challenging problem of recovering the second-order optical nonlinearity depth profile of thin films is addressed. When compared with the level of the prior art, our solutions to this problem are a *breakthrough*. We divide our solutions into two main categories: (1) interferometric techniques, and (2) non-interferometric techniques. The interferometric techniques, discussed in Section 3.2, enable analytical recovery of the nonlinearity depth profile, whereas the non-interferometric techniques, discussed in Section 3.3, rely on iterative recovery algorithms based on minimum phase functions. The clear advantage of the non-interferometric approach is its simplicity and flexibility, both experimentally and computationally, together with the lack of artificial "ringing" in the output results. However, as further discussed in Section 3.3, it is limited to special class of nonlinear materials, such as poled glasses or sputtered thin films. The interferometric approach, though being more difficult to implement experimentally, has the advantage of being able to recover the depth profile of all possible nonlinear thin films, without exceptions. Historically, the analytical recovery techniques based on spectral interferometry were developed first, which led to the discovery and independent confirmation of the non-interferometric iterative approach.

3.2 ANALYTICAL CHARACTERIZATION TOOLS USING SPECTRAL INTERFEROMETRY

In this section, three powerful analytical techniques that enable to uniquely retrieve the second-order nonlinearity profile of thin films are discussed.[2-4] These techniques all make use of Maker-fringe (MF) measurements,[7] which involve focusing a fundamental laser beam onto the nonlinear film under test and measuring the second-harmonic (SH) power generated in the nonlinear region as a function of the incidence angle of the fundamental beam. As will be discussed in detail later on, the data provided by this measurement, also called the MF curve, carries crucial information about the nonlinearity profile. Specifically, the MF curve is proportional to the square of the Fourier transform (FT) magnitude of the nonlinearity profile $d(z)$, where z is the direction normal to the surface of the film. However, this measurement does not provide the phase of the FT, which cannot be directly measured in a simple manner. With such a classical MF measurement, it is therefore impossible to invert the FT and retrieve $d(z)$ uniquely. Our analytical techniques[1-4] are based on the observation that by recording the MF curves of two nonlinear films sandwiched together, the fundamental and SH waves interfere in the two films in such a way that the FT phase of both samples is now embedded in the measured MF curve. It is then possible to process this MF curve to recover these two FT phases, and thus to reconstruct the full complex FT of the two nonlinearity profiles. These two FTs can then be easily inverted to retrieve the nonlinearity profiles of both films.

In this chapter, a detailed description of the mathematical foundations of these three analytical techniques,[2-4] pointing in particular to the relationship between these techniques and their relative merits and disadvantages will be discussed. Furthermore, we will present an error analysis of each technique to estimate the error in the recovered profiles. In Section 3.2.1, we discuss the classical Maker-fringe (MF) technique and how a measured MF curve is processed to retrieve the FT amplitude of the nonlinearity profile. In Section 3.2.2, the theory for recovering $d(z)$ using the most general of the three techniques (the two-sample technique) is described. The other two analytical techniques (the twin-sample and the reference-sample techniques), which can be considered as special cases are discussed in Appendix A. The error analysis of these techniques is presented in Section 3.2.3. In Section 3.2.4, we describe an experimental demonstration of all three techniques, and show a comparison between inferred profiles. A further discussion on these analytical techniques will also be given in Section 3.2.5.

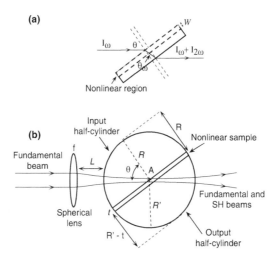

Fig. 1. (a) Generation of SH from a nonlinear region of width W, as a function of incidence angle, θ, (b) cylinder-assisted Maker-fringe set-up.

3.2.1 PROPERTIES AND LIMITATIONS OF THE CLASSICAL MAKER-FRINGE TECHNIQUE

The Maker-fringe measurement is the most commonly used techniques to measure the second-order nonlinearity of thin films.[7] A fundamental laser beam of wavelength λ, typically in the near infrared, is focused onto a wafer that has a second-order optical nonlinearity at an incidence angle θ (see Fig. 1(a)), and the second-harmonic (SH) power generated by frequency doubling within the nonlinear region of this sample is recorded at the output of the wafer as a function of θ. Due to refraction at the input face of the sample, the internal propagation angle of the fundamental beam inside the nonlinear film becomes θ_ω, given by $\sin\theta = n_\omega \sin\theta_\omega$, where n_ω is the refractive index of the film at λ, and $\omega = 2\pi c/\lambda$ is the angular frequency of the fundamental wave, where c is the speed of light. To remain general, we consider the situation where only a portion of the wafer is optically nonlinear, as occurs for example in a poled silica wafer (in which case the nonlinear region is confined to a few tens of microns below the surface) or a thin film of nonlinear organic material deposited on an optically "linear" wafer. If W is the thickness of the nonlinear region, the effective propagation length of the beam through the nonlinear region is $W/\cos\theta_\omega$. Therefore, as the incidence angle increases, so does the path of the fundamental beam through the nonlinear region. Due to the finite dispersion between the fundamental and SH signals, as these two signals get in and out of phase, the direction of energy coupling changes, and the amount of generated SH power oscillates with the angle θ_ω. These oscillations are known as Maker fringes.[7] The quantity that is typically plotted is the second-harmonic generation (SHG) efficiency as a function of the internal propagation angle θ_ω, i.e., $\eta(\theta_\omega) = I_{2\omega}(\theta_\omega)/I_\omega^2$, where I_ω and $I_{2\omega}$ are the intensities of the fundamental beam at the input and the SH beam at the output of the sample, respectively (see Fig. 1(a)). The SHG efficiency is described theoretically by integrating the second-order nonlinear coefficient profile of the thin film $d(z)$ along z:[1,2]

$$\eta(\theta_\omega) = K(\theta_\omega) \cdot \left| \int_{-\infty}^{\infty} d(z) \cdot \exp(j\Delta k(\theta_\omega)z) \cdot dz \right|^2 \qquad (1)$$

The nonlinear coefficient of Eq. (1), $d(z)$, can vary depending on the orientation of the nonlinear material and the polarization of the fundamental and second-harmonic waves. For poled silica, for a TM polarized fundamental wave, $d = d_{33}$ and for a TE polarized fundamental wave $d = d_{31}$, where $d_{33} = 3\,d_{31}$. [9] Furthermore, $K(\theta_\omega)$ of Eq. (1) is a known proportionality constant that accounts in particular for the Fresnel reflection loss of each wave at the input and output faces of the sample. [9] $\Delta k(\theta_\omega)$ is the wave-vector mismatch between the two beams in the z direction, given by $\Delta k(\theta_\omega) = \dfrac{4\pi}{\lambda}(n_\omega \cos\theta_\omega - n_{2\omega}\cos\theta_{2\omega})$, where $n_{2\omega}$ and $\theta_{2\omega}$ are the refractive index and the internal propagation angle at the SH frequency 2ω, respectively. When the dispersion between the two waves is small, $\Delta k(\theta_\omega)$ can be approximated by $\Delta k(\theta_\omega) \approx \dfrac{4\pi}{\lambda}\dfrac{n_\omega - n_{2\omega}}{\cos\theta_{2\omega}} \approx \dfrac{4\pi}{\lambda}\dfrac{n_\omega - n_{2\omega}}{\cos\theta_\omega}$. Note that this approximation is generally not valid for large incidence angles.

The integral in Eq. (1) is the Fourier transform $D(f)$ of the nonlinearity profile $d(z)$, where the spatial frequency is defined as $f = \pm\left|\dfrac{\Delta k(\theta_\omega)}{2\pi}\right|$. Therefore, the quantity that is measured in a classical MF method is the spectrum of the square of the amplitude of the FT of $d(z)$, i.e., $|D(f)|^2$. Again, since this measurement does not provide the phase of $D(f)$, it is generally not possible, without additional data, to invert $D(f)$ and recover $d(z)$ from this measurement alone.

A second consequence of Eq. (1) is that the inverse Fourier transform (IFT) of the MF curve is the auto-correlation of $d(z)$, since $IFT\left\{|D(f)|^2\right\} = C(z) = d(z)\otimes d(z) = d(z)*d(-z)$, where '$\otimes$' and '$*$' stand for the correlation and convolution operations, respectively. As demonstrated in Appendix B, this auto-correlation function $C(z)$ can provide an estimate of the depth of the profile $d(z)$. However, $C(z)$ is not sufficient to uniquely determine the physical function $d(z)$. This limitation has the same mathematical origin as the missing FT phase mentioned in the previous paragraph.

A third point is that the spatial frequency f depends on the cosine of the internal propagation angle. This angle can be measured at most between 0 and 90°. Consequently, the measured frequencies $f = \dfrac{2}{\lambda}(n_\omega \cos\theta_\omega - n_{2\omega}\cos\theta_{2\omega})$ provided by this measurement are strictly negative, which means that an MF measurement can only provide the spectrum of $|D(f)|$ over half of the frequency space. However, since $d(z)$ is real,

$|D(f)| = |D(-f)|$, which means that the other half of the FT amplitude spectrum is also known. Therefore, in spite of this limitation, an MF measurement provides $|D(f)|$ in both halves of the frequency space.

A fourth point is that in practice, total internal reflection (TIR) at the output face of the wafer limits θ_ω to a value smaller than 90°. For instance, in poled silica, TIR occurs at $\theta_\omega \approx 43°$. Above this angle the second-harmonic field is totally reflected at the output face and the detected power artificially drops to zero. The FT information above 43° is thus lost. Fresnel reflection losses at the input face of the sample also limit the maximum achievable incidence angle. These two limitations can be avoided by placing prisms, spherical lenses or cylindrical lenses on both sides of the wafer (see Fig. 1(b)), which allows the measurement of MF curves up to internal angles approaching ~90°.[5] A detailed discussion regarding some significant advantages of using cylindrical lenses is given in Appendix C. These approaches are important to measure $|D(f)|$ up to as high a frequency as possible.

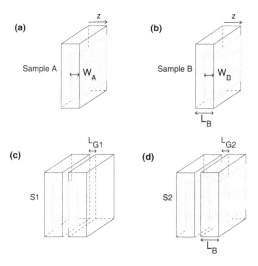

Fig. 2. (a), (b), (c), (d) Sample A, Sample B, S1 and S2 configurations, respectively, with the corresponding nonlinear regions shown in gray.

A final and rather crucial point is that an MF measurement fails to provide both the DC and the high-frequency end portions of $|D(f)|$. Even when the SHG efficiency is measured over the full range of internal angles θ_ω (0° to 90°), the spatial frequencies that are actually measured range only from $f_{min} = \left| \dfrac{\Delta k(\theta_\omega = 0°)}{2\pi} \right| = 2\left| \dfrac{n_\omega - n_{2\omega}}{\lambda} \right|$ to

$f_{max} = \left| \dfrac{\Delta k(\theta_\omega = 90°)}{2\pi} \right| = 2 \dfrac{\sqrt{n_{2\omega}^2 - n_\omega^2}}{\lambda}$, i.e., $f_{min} > 0$ and $f_{max} < \infty$. For example, for a

typical poled silica sample characterized at 1064 nm, $f_{min} \approx 2 \times 10^4 \, m^{-1}$ and $f_{max} \approx 3.4 \times 10^5 \, m^{-1}$. Thus an MF measurement can only provide a finite (albeit large) portion of the $|D(f)|$ spectrum, namely over the frequency intervals [-f_{max}, -f_{min}] and [f_{min}, f_{max}], and never over the full frequency range ([$-\infty, +\infty$]). We show in this work that the missing DC and high-frequency portions of $|D(f)|$ can be recovered uniquely from the measured portion of the spectrum by using one of several well-known mathematical extrapolation techniques. To show proof of principle, we used the Papoulis-Gerchberg (PG) algorithm.[12-14] The details of this iterative method can be found in Appendix B, including numerical examples that illustrate its accuracy in the context of MF spectra.

3.2.2 THEORY FOR ANALYTICAL RECOVERY OF $d(z)$

In this section, we present the theory for determining the nonlinearity profile of thin films using a general two-sample technique, which involves measuring the MF curve of a structure formed by sandwiching two different nonlinear samples in two different configurations (Fig. 2).[3] The interference between the second-harmonic signals generated from the two samples carries the information to determine the phase of the FT. The special cases of nominally identical samples (the twin-sample technique[2]) and of one sample having a known nonlinearity profile (the reference-sample technique[4]) are analyzed separately in Appendix A. In each case, a numerical simulation of the recovery of $d(z)$, including the application of the PG algorithm, is presented.

3.2.2.1 The most general case: The two-sample method

For the most general treatment of the problem, we consider two different wafers A and B with respective unknown nonlinearity profiles $d_A(z)$ and $d_B(z)$. These profiles are assumed to be different, although this condition is actually not necessary.

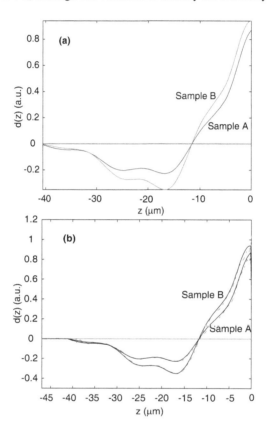

Fig. 3. (a) Arbitrarily chosen theoretical nonlinearity profiles for samples A and B, (b) the result of the recovery (dashed curves) for samples A and B using the two-sample method. The solid curves are the initially assumed theoretical profiles, the same as shown in (a).

We assume that both profiles are uniform in the plane of the wafer and have a finite extent in the z direction. By definition, the nonlinearity is confined to the negative z space, i.e., $d_A(z) = 0$ for $z > 0$ and $z < -W_A$ and $d_B(z) = 0$ for $z > 0$ and $z < -W_B$, where $z =$

0 is the surface of each sample and W_A and W_B are the depths of the nonlinear regions of samples A and B, respectively (see Figs. 2(a) and 2(b)).

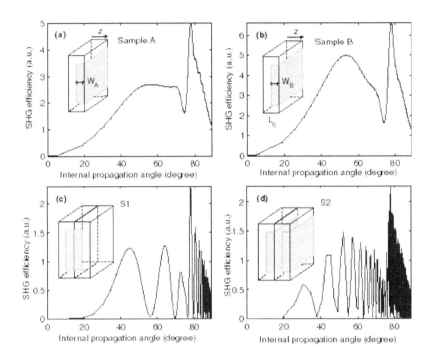

Fig. 4. (a), (b), (c), (d) MF curves of sample A, sample B, S1 and S2 configurations, respectively, theoretically computed from the two profiles shown in Fig. 3(a).

Our aim is to determine both $d_A(z)$ and $d_B(z)$ uniquely, using the MF measurements of two sandwich structures formed by assembling these two samples in appropriate configurations. The first structure, labeled S1, is formed by mating the $z = 0$ surface of sample A with the $z = 0$ surface of sample B, as shown in Fig. 2(c). The second structure (S2) is formed by mating the $z = 0$ surface of sample A with the opposite surface of sample B, as shown in Fig. 2(d). In both structures, an index-matching gel or liquid is placed between the samples to avoid TIR at their interface. For reasons explained further on, it may also be advantageous to insert an optically linear silica spacer between the samples. The respective separations between the mated surfaces are then L_{G1} (Fig. 2(c)) and L_{G2} (Fig. 2(d)). In the absence of spacers, L_{G1} and L_{G2} represent the thickness of the index-matching layers. The MF curves of these two structures are measured using the conventional MF-measurement set-up shown in Fig. C4 of Appendix C. The fundamental beam was supplied by a 1064-nm Q-switched Nd:YAG laser (~30-ns full-width at half maximum pulses with a maximum energy of ~750 µJ) operated at 1 kHz. The beam was first passed through a half-wave plate to align its polarization with respect to the sample (transverse magnetic), then focused onto the sample with a ~15-cm focal-length lens. The sample was sandwiched between two half-cylinders to avoid TIR.[5] The signals emerging from the sample were recollimated with a lens, and the fundamental beam was eliminated with a 1064-nm high reflector, IR filters, and a 532-nm spike filter. The SHG pulse was finally detected with a photo-multiplier tube (PMT).

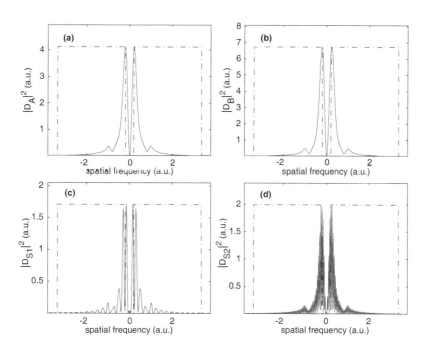

Fig. 5. (a), (b), (c), (d) Square of the magnitude of the FT spectrum of the nonlinearity profiles of sample A, sample B, S1 and S2 configurations, respectively. The dashed rectangular curves denote the frequency range that the MF measurements provide.

To illustrate the steps in the data processing that lead to the retrieval of $d_A(z)$ and $d_B(z)$, and to demonstrate the accuracy of the two-sample technique, in the following treatment, we use the two arbitrarily chosen nonlinearity profiles $d_A(z)$ and $d_B(z)$ plotted in Fig. 3(a). Note that there is nothing special about these two profiles, and any two randomly selected profiles will yield comparable quantitative results.

To understand the role of the MF curves of S1 and S2, consider first the classical MF measurements of individual samples A and B. As discussed in Section 2, these MF curves are proportional to the square of the magnitude of the FT of $d_A(z)$ and $d_B(z)$, respectively, i.e.,

$$MF_A(f) = |D_A(f)|^2 \quad (2)$$

$$MF_B(f) = |D_B(f)|^2 \quad (3)$$

where $|D_A(f)|$ and $|D_B(f)|$ are the magnitude of the FT of $d_A(z)$ and $d_B(z)$, respectively. The proportionality constant is the same for all measured MF curves, and for simplicity this constant is not shown.

These two MF curves, computed numerically for the two profiles of Fig. 3(a), are plotted in Figs. 4(a) and 4(b). Once again, these classical MF measurements do not provide the FT phases of $d_A(z)$ and $d_B(z)$, $\phi_A(f)$ and $\phi_B(f)$. However, in the MF measurements of S1 and S2, even though only the angular spectra of SH powers are recorded, this information contains both $\phi_A(f)$ and $\phi_B(f)$. To validate this key point, let us first analyze the MF curve of sandwich structure S1. To provide physical insight, and without loss of generality, we will pursue this discussion for the special case of poled silica. The $z = 0$ planes are defined here as the surfaces of samples A and B where the anode was placed during poling. The nonlinearity profile of sandwich S1 can be written as $d_{S1}(z) = d_A(z) - d_B(-z + L_{G1})$. Since sample B is flipped 180° to mate with the $z = 0$ surface of sample A, as far as the interacting optical beams traversing sample B are concerned, the sign of the nonlinearity profile of sample B is reversed, which explains the minus sign in this expression.

The MF curve of S1 is proportional to the square of the magnitude of the FT of $d_{S1}(z)$:

$$MF_{S1} = |D_{S1}|^2 = |D_A|^2 + |D_B|^2 - 2|D_A||D_B|\cos(\phi_A + \phi_B + \phi_1) \quad (4)$$

where $\phi_1(f) = 2\pi f L_{G1}$ is a phase term that accounts for the phase delay of the fundamental beam through the spacer. All quantities in Eq. 4 depend on the spatial frequency, but this dependence has been dropped for convenience.

Similarly, the nonlinearity profile of S2 can be written as $d_{S2}(z) = d_A(z) + d_B(z - L)$, where $L = L_B + L_{G2}$ and L_B is the thickness of sample B. The MF curve of S2 can thus be expressed as:

$$MF_{S2} = |D_{S2}|^2 = |D_A|^2 + |D_B|^2 + 2|D_A||D_B|\cos(\phi_A - \phi_B + \phi_2) \quad (5)$$

where $\phi_2(f) = 2\pi f L$. Note that alternatively, sandwich S2 can be replaced by a new sandwich structure (S3), where both samples are flipped 180°. It can be shown that the MF curve of S3 also contains the phase information $\phi_A - \phi_B$, and therefore can be used as an alternative to S2. We selected S2 simply because the distance between nonlinear regions is smaller than in S3 (at least in the case of poled silica samples), which means that the MF curve of this S2 configuration does not oscillate as much and is therefore somewhat easier to measure experimentally.

The MF curves of S1 and S2, computed for the two profiles of Fig. 3(a), assuming $L_{G1} = L_{G2} = 40$ μm and $L_B = 150$ μm, are shown in Figs. 4(c) and 4(d), respectively. The MF curve of S2 exhibits rapid oscillations because the separation between nonlinear regions is fairly large ($L = L_B + L_{G2} = 190$ μm), which implies a large phase term $\phi_2(f) = 2\pi f L$ in Eq. (5). The squares of the FT amplitudes $|D_A(f)|^2$, $|D_B(f)|^2$, $|D_{S1}(f)|^2$ and $|D_{S2}(f)|^2$, which were calculated from the four MF curves of Fig. (4), are shown in Figs. 5(a)-(d). As explained previously, in an actual MF measurement only the portions [-f_{max}, -f_{min}] and [f_{min}, f_{max}] of the frequency space would actually be obtained. These two ranges are outlined in Fig. 5 by the dashed rectangles. In other words, had the spectra

MF_{S1} and MF_{S2} been obtained by measurement, only the portions of the spectra within these rectangles would be known at this point. In this numerical example, the missing DC and high-frequency-end portions of each spectrum were recovered using the PG algorithm,[14] as discussed in Section 2, with an average error less than 0.06% (see Appendix B). This nearly perfect recovery is also shown in Fig. 5, which plots both the theoretical and the recovered spectra.

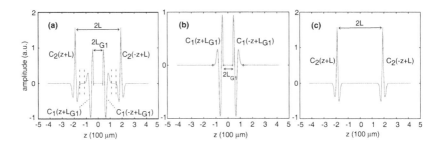

Fig. 6. (a) IFT of $|D_{S2}|^2 - |D_{S1}|^2$, (b) IFT of $-|D_{S1}|^2 + |D_A|^2 + |D_B|^2$, (c) IFT of $|D_{S2}|^2 - |D_A|^2 - |D_B|^2$.

The profiles $d_A(z)$ and $d_B(z)$ are recovered from the MF curves of S1 and S2 as follows. The first step is to take the IFT of the difference $|D_{S2}(f)|^2 - |D_{S1}(f)|^2$. This IFT is composed of two terms, namely $IFT\{2|D_A||D_B|\cos(\phi_A - \phi_B + \phi_2)\}$ and $IFT\{2|D_A||D_B|\cos(\phi_A + \phi_B + \phi_1)\}$. Using basic properties of Fourier transforms, these two terms can be expressed as:

$$IFT\{2|D_A||D_B|\cos(\phi_A + \phi_B + \phi_1)\} = C_1(-z + L_{G1}) + C_1(z + L_{G1}) \quad (6)$$

$$IFT\{2|D_A||D_B|\cos(\phi_A - \phi_B + \phi_2)\} = C_2(-z + L) + C_2(z + L) \quad (7)$$

where $C_1(z)$ and $C_2(z)$ are the convolution functions $C_1(z) = d_A(z) * d_B(z)$ and $C_2(z) = d_A(z) * d_B(-z)$, respectively. $IFT\{|D_{S2}(f)|^2 - |D_{S1}(f)|^2\}$, calculated from the spectra $|D_{S1}(f)|^2$ of Fig. 5(c) and $|D_{S2}(f)|^2$ of Fig. 5(d), is plotted in Fig. 6(a). This figure shows that the spectra $C_1(z + L_{G1})$ and $C_2(z + L)$ do not overlap in space, and they can therefore be recovered individually. The second step in the data processing is to recover $C_1(z+L_{G1})$ and $C_2(z+L)$ from this graph (Fig. 6(a)). The third step is to simply shift these recovered spectra in space by L_{G1} and L, respectively, to obtain $C_1(z)$ and $C_2(z)$. This step is straightforward, since L_{G1} and L are measurable quantities. A further discussion on the measurement of L_{G1} and L will be presented later on. The fourth step is to compute the FTs of $C_1(z)$ and $C_2(z)$, which are equal to $|D_A| \cdot |D_B| \cdot \exp(j[\phi_A + \phi_B])$ and $|D_A| \cdot |D_B| \cdot \exp(j[\phi_A - \phi_B])$, respectively, and then to add and subtract the phases of these two FTs to obtain $\phi_A(f)$ and $\phi_B(f)$, i.e., the phases of the FT of $d_A(z)$ and $d_B(z)$. This is an important result: the phase spectra of the Fourier transforms have been recovered, which would not have been possible with classical MF measurement systems. In the fifth step, the phases $\phi_A(f)$ and $\phi_B(f)$, together with the FT amplitude of $C_1(z)$ (or $C_2(z)$), i.e., the product $|D_A| \cdot |D_B|$, are inserted in either Eq. (4) or Eq. (5) to obtain $|D_A|^2 + |D_B|^2$, which, combined with $|D_A| \cdot |D_B|$, yields the FT amplitudes $|D_A|$ and $|D_B|$. The final step is to take the IFT of the recovered quantities $|D_A(f)| \exp(j\phi_A(f))$ and $|D_B(f)| \exp(j\phi_B(f))$ to obtain $d_A(z)$ and $d_B(z)$. This algorithm requires the measurement of two MF curves, namely MF_{S1} and MF_{S2}. Since in the end it provides two originally unknown nonlinearity profiles, this technique requires the same number of measurements per profile as a classical MF measurement.

As pointed above, this data processing algorithm is possible only if the spectra $C_1(z+L_{G1})$ and $C_2(z+L)$ do not overlap. It can be shown mathematically that this requirement is satisfied provided the various thicknesses involved in S2 satisfy the condition $L = L_B + L_{G2} > 2W_B + W_A + L_{G1}$. For any given samples A and B, this condition can always be satisfied by choosing a sufficiently large L_B, i.e., either a thick enough nonlinear sample, or, if this is not possible, by using a large enough L_{G2}, i.e., a thick enough spacer. This requirement explains the possible need for spacers stated above. For special cases where choosing a thick enough nonlinear sample and/or spacer is not a preferred option, the two convolutions spectra do overlap, and recovery of $d_A(z)$ and $d_B(z)$ using this algorithm is no longer possible. However, recovery can still be performed by using additional information, namely by measuring $MF_A(f)$ and $MF_B(f)$.

The algorithm then involves taking the IFT of two linear combinations of the three MF curves, namely:

$$IFT\left\{\frac{1}{2}|D_{S1}|^2 + |D_A|^2 + |D_B|^2\right\} = IFT\left\{2|D_A||D_B|\cos(\phi_A + \phi_B + \phi_1)\right\}$$
$$= C_1(-z + L_{G1}) + C_1(z + L_{G1})$$ (8)

$$IFT\left\{|D_{S2}|^2 - |D_A|^2 - |D_B|^2\right\} = IFT\left\{2|D_A||D_B|\cos(\phi_A - \phi_B + \phi_2)\right\}$$
$$= C_2(-z + L) + C_2(z + L)$$ (9)

The IFT in Eq. (8) is the sum of two convolutions, one centered at $+L_{G1}$ and confined to the $z > 0$ space, the other centered at $-L_{G1}$ and confined to the $z < 0$ space (see Fig. 6(b)). Therefore, without any spatial overlap the convolution $C_1(z + L_{G1})$ can easily be recovered. Similarly, the IFT in Eq. (9) is the sum of two convolutions confined in different portions of space (see Fig. 6(c)), and the convolution $C_2(z + L)$ is easily recovered. The rest of the recovery algorithm is the same as described above for the $L = L_B + L_{G2} > 2W_B + W_A + L_{G1}$ case.

In practice, retrieving $C_1(z)$ and $C_2(z)$ from $C_1(z + L_{G1})$ and $C_2(z + L)$ during the third step of the algorithm requires the knowledge of L_{G1} and $L = L_B + L_{G2}$. Where applicable, these two lengths can be directly measured. However, this measurement is not actually necessary, because both L_{G1} and L can be determined from the measured spectra MF_{S1} and MF_{S2}. In Eqs. (4) and (5), the terms $\phi_1(f) = 2\pi f L_{G1}$ and $\phi_2(f) = 2\pi f L$ are modulation terms. Since $MF_{S1} \le (|D_A| + |D_B|)^2$ (see Eq. (4)) and $MF_{S2} \le (|D_A| + |D_B|)^2$ (see Eq. (5)), the term $(|D_A| + |D_B|)^2$ is an envelope for these modulation terms. Therefore, under the slowly varying envelope approximation, L_{G1} and $L = L_B + L_{G2}$ can be determined from the period of the maxima in the MF_{S1} and MF_{S2} spectra, respectively. The validity of this method can easily be verified by applying it to the MF curves of Figs. 4(c) and 4(d), which yields $L_{G1} = 40.22$ μm and $L = 190.49$ μm, respectively. The corresponding theoretical values for these thicknesses are 40 μm and 190 μm, respectively, so the error in the values recovered by this process is less than 0.6%. A second method for determining L_{G1} and L is to look at the IFT of $|D_{S2}|^2 - |D_{S1}|^2$, shown in Fig. 6(a). Since by definition $C_1(z = 0) = 0$, and the gap in Fig. 6(a) around $z = 0$ is equal to $2L_{G1}$, L_{G1} can easily be determined from the gap as $L_{G1} \approx 39.27 \, \mu m$, with an error of only 1.8%.

Note that errors in L and L_{G1} are inconsequential. To prove this point, let ε_1 and ε_2 be the errors made in the determination of L_{G1} and L, respectively. The recovered convolution functions $C_1(z)$ and $C_2(z)$ will then be $C_1(z+\varepsilon_1)$ and $C_2(z+\varepsilon_2)$, respectively. The FT of $C_1(z+\varepsilon_1)$ and $C_2(z+\varepsilon_2)$ become $|D_A| \cdot |D_B| \cdot \exp\left(j[\phi_A + \phi_B - 2\pi f \varepsilon_1]\right)$ and $|D_A| \cdot |D_B| \cdot \exp\left(j[\phi_A - \phi_B - 2\pi f \varepsilon_2]\right)$. When adding and subtracting the FT phases of $C_1(z+\varepsilon_1)$ and $C_2(z+\varepsilon_2)$ in the fourth step of the recovery, the FT phases of $d_A(z)$ and $d_B(z)$ are $\phi_A - \pi f(\varepsilon_1+\varepsilon_2)$ and $\phi_B - \pi f(\varepsilon_1-\varepsilon_2)$. The recovered nonlinearity profiles thus become $d_A(z+\frac{\varepsilon_1+\varepsilon_2}{2})$ and $d_B(z+\frac{\varepsilon_1-\varepsilon_2}{2})$. Therefore, errors in the knowledge of L and L_{G1} cause an error in the relative location of the nonlinear region within the wafer, but have no impact on the shape and magnitude of the recovered profiles. Furthermore, depending on the relative signs of ε_1 and ε_2, for either $d_A(z)$ or $d_B(z)$ the errors can at least partially cancel each other.

To evaluate the performance of this algorithm, we applied it to the two nonlinearity profiles $d_A(z)$ and $d_B(z)$ of Fig. 3(a). In a first step, using these two spectra, we computed numerically the MF spectra MF_{S1} and MF_{S2} of sandwich structures S1 and S2. Aside from experimental errors and noise, we would have obtained these same spectra had we actually measured the MF curves of the sandwich structures S1 and S2 formed with the two unknown samples. We then applied the above algorithm to MF_{S1} and MF_{S2} to retrieve these two profiles and compared them to the actual profiles of Fig. 3(a). As can be seen in Fig. 3(a), both samples have the same profile depth i.e., $W_A = W_B = 40.6$ μm. The intermediate steps of this recovery have been previously discussed in relation to Figs. 4, 5, and 6.

The recovered profiles of samples A and B are shown as dashed curves in Fig. 3(b), together with the original assumed profiles (solid curves) for comparison. In both cases, the recovery is close to perfect. The mean square error in the recovered profiles, defined as $\dfrac{\int |d(z) - \hat{d}(z)|^2 \, dz}{\int |d(z)|^2 \cdot dz}$, where $d(z)$ and $\hat{d}(z)$ are the theoretical and the recovered nonlinearity profiles, respectively, is 0.28% and 0.21% for $d_A(z)$ and $d_B(z)$, respectively. The error analysis presented above showed the recovered profiles to be $d_A(z + \dfrac{\varepsilon_1 + \varepsilon_2}{2})$ and

$d_B(z + \dfrac{\varepsilon_1 - \varepsilon_2}{2})$. Since ε_1 = 40.22 - 40 = 0.22 μm and ε_2 = 190.49 - 190 = 0.49 μm, we expect better recovery for $d_B(z)$ than for $d_A(z)$, as actually observed in Fig. 3.

3.2.3 ERROR ANALYSIS

Several sources introduce errors in the measured MF curves of nonlinear samples, and thus in the recovered profiles. In this section, we investigate the main sources of error, calculate their quantitative impact on the accuracy of the recovered profile, and propose various methods to improve this accuracy.

The first source of error arises from diffraction: as a result of the finite size of the fundamental beam, a range of internal angles is excited in the nonlinear region. Each incremental angle within this range excites its own Maker fringe curve. At small incidence angles, the MF curve is generally weakly dependent on angle (see for example Fig. 4); thus, all these incremental MF curves are nearly identical and simply add into a single curve. At high angles, however, the Maker fringes generally oscillate strongly and these incremental MF curves differ markedly, and the detector records an average of these curves. This portion of the curve is then not the actual MF curve but the average of the actual curve over the range of excited internal angles. If the MF curve oscillates several times within this range, these oscillations are completely washed out. This effect worsens as the incidence angle approaches 90°. It also worsens for thicker nonlinear regions, which produce MF curves that oscillate more rapidly. This is particularly true for sandwich S2, which comprises two nonlinear regions that are fairly far apart.

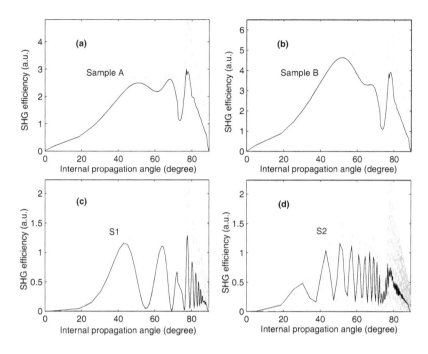

Fig. 7. (a), (b), (c), (d) Distorted MF curves (solid curves) for the error analysis of the recovery techniques, corresponding to sample A, sample B, S1 and S2 configurations, respectively. The dashed gray curves are the original error-free theoretical MF curves for the same samples.

The second source of error is amplitude errors in the MF curves due to measurement uncertainties such as laser power fluctuations or PMT noise. It turns out that this contribution is smaller than the error due to diffraction, so in this study we will ignore it.

The third source of error occurs when the maximum-recorded internal angle is significantly less than 90°. This limitation lowers f_{max} and thus increases the frequency range over which the data needs to be extrapolated using the PG algorithm, rather than measured. Although this algorithm is quite accurate, it does introduce a finite error, especially when the range of measured angles is small (lower f_{max}). This is not the case for poled silica: for this material it is straightforward to achieve good index matching, thus we can virtually eliminate TIR and achieve a maximum internal angle very close to

90° (~89.6° has been demonstrated[5]). However, for some nonlinear materials, in particular materials with higher refractive indices or high birefringence, avoiding TIR may be more difficult and this effect may be significant.

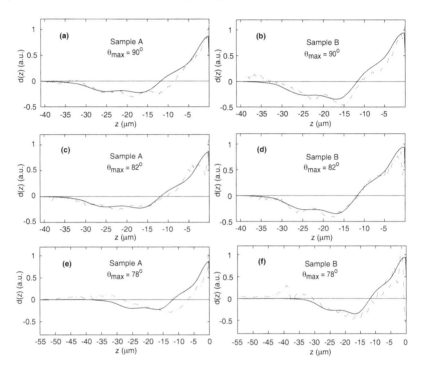

Fig. 8. Result of the recovery (dashed curves) using the two-sample technique and the distorted MF curves of Fig. 7 for (a), (b) θ_{max} = 90°; (c), (d) θ_{max} = 82°; (e), (f) θ_{max} = 78°, for sample A and sample B, respectively. The solid curves are the theoretically assumed nonlinearity profiles.

To simulate the effects of the errors due to the diffraction and the lower f_{max} on the accuracy of the recovered profiles, we used the more general two-sample method (see Section 3.2.2.1). This analysis can be readily extended to the other two techniques and yields similar results. For the purpose of illustration, in our simulations we will again use the two nonlinearity profiles of Fig. 3(a) and the same parameter values as in Section 3.2.2.1. The error-free MF curves (MF_A, MF_B, MF_{S1} and MF_{S2}) and the two profiles recovered in the absence of diffraction were discussed in Section 3.2.2.1 (see Figs. 4 and 3(b), and are reproduced as dash-doted curves in Fig. 7.

To simulate the effects of diffraction realistically, for each internal propagation angle θ_ω we multiplied the error-free MF curve by a rectangular window of width $\delta\theta_\omega$, and replaced the original value of the MF curve at θ_ω by the average of the MF curve over this window. Since diffraction effects worsen at higher angles, roughly as $1/\cos(\theta_\omega)$, the width $\delta\theta_\omega$ was taken to increase as $1/\cos(\theta_\omega)$. The result of this process is shown in Figs. 7(a) through (d). In each frame, the dashed curve is the original error-free MF curve and the solid curve is the same curve after the diffraction-induced error has been added. This error has little effect on MF_A (Fig. 7(a)) and MF_B (Fig. 7(b)) because these curves oscillate slowly. The effect is considerably larger in MF_{S_1} (Fig. 7(c)) and MF_{S_2} (Fig. 7(d)) at large angles, where oscillations are rapid. In this example, the mean square error introduced by diffraction, across the whole angular spectrum, is ~20% for MF_1 and MF_2, ~30% for MF_{S1}, and ~40% for MF_{S2}.

From these "noisy" MF curves, W_A, W_B, L_{Gl}, and L were estimated to be 39 μm, 36 μm, 41.8 μm, and 190.7 μm, with respective errors of ~5%, ~12%, ~5% and ~0.5%. The nonlinearity profiles of samples A and B, recovered by applying the two-sample method, are shown as the dashed curves in Figs. 8(a) and 8(b), respectively. These curves were calculated for a maximum measured internal propagation angle of 90°. For comparison, the exact original profiles are shown as solid curves. For this maximum recorded angle, the recovered curves do show small departures from the original profiles. The mean square difference between the two profiles is 10% for $d_A(z)$ and 8% for $d_B(z)$. These figures show that the error in the profile is much smaller than the error in the Maker fringe curve (in this example ~40% in MF_{S2}), i.e., these recovery methods are quite tolerant of errors in the measured MF curves. Once again, since $\varepsilon_1 \times \varepsilon_2 > 0$, i.e., ε_1 and ε_2 have the same sign, the theory predicts a smaller error on $d_B(z)$, as observed (see end of section 3.2.2.1).

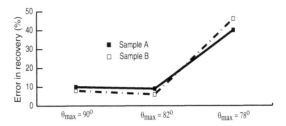

Fig. 9. The mean square error in the recovered nonlinearity profiles using the two-sample technique and the distorted MF curves of Fig. 7 as a function of θ_{max}.

To evaluate the effect on the accuracy of the retrieved profiles of the third source of error (maximum achievable angle less than 90°), the "noisy" MF curves of Fig. 7 were truncated at angles above $\theta_{max} \approx 82°$, as again might occur as a result of TIR due to an index mismatch. The recovered profiles of samples A and B are plotted in Figs. 8(c) and 8(d), respectively. The overall agreement is now slightly better, with average errors of 9% for $d_A(z)$ and 6% for $d_B(z)$. If the maximum recorded angle is lowered by just 4° (to 78°), the errors increase to 40% and 46% (see Figs. 8(e) and 8(f)). The dependence of the error on θ_{max} is plotted in Fig. 9. It shows clearly the existence of an optimum maximum angle θ_{opt} that minimizes the error in the profile. This optimum angle depends on the noise level and on the divergence of the fundamental beam. For the parameter values used in our simulations, the optimum angle is $\theta_{opt} \approx 82°$. An optimum angle exists because if θ_{max} is too low, fewer data points are available in the MF curves to extrapolate the missing higher frequency components with the PG algorithm, and the latter introduces a larger error in the recovered profile. On the other hand, if θ_{max} is too high, the error in the measured MF curve at the highest angles due to diffraction increases and the recovered profile accuracy gets worse. In other words, because of diffraction, it is more accurate to obtain the high-angle portion of the MF curves (above θ_{opt}) with the PG algorithm than with an actual measurement.

The overall conclusion of this section is that all three analytical IFT techniques[2-4] are quite tolerant of errors in the measured MF curves: the average error in the recovered profile is about 4 times smaller than the mean error in the measured MF curve.

With a suitable choice of the maximum recorded angle, the error in the recovered profiles due to the two main sources of error is quite small, of the order of 8% in our example.

3.2.4 EXPERIMENTAL RESULTS

In this section, the analytical tools described so far will be experimentally demonstrated on thermally poled silica samples. Before we present the recovery results in this material system, let us first introduce the basics of poled silica in the next section.

3.2.4.1 THERMALLY POLED SILICA

Poled glass has been an active area of research over the last few years because of the prospect of using this nonlinear material for integrated electro-optic phase and amplitude modulators or parametric oscillators.[1-6,8-11,15-26] Poled silica-based glasses are particularly appropriate for these applications because they exhibit low loss, broad transmission bands, and high optical damage threshold, and are compatible with current fiber optic technology. One of the main limitations of this material, however, is that its nonlinear coefficient is low, with a peak second-order optical nonlinear coefficient d_{33} of only ~0.8 pm/V (compared to ~30 pm/V for LiNbO$_3$).[2] As a result, all poled-glass devices reported to date require high voltages and/or long lengths.[16]

Thermal poling is one of the most commonly used techniques to induce a permanent second-order nonlinearity in silica, normally a centro-symmetric material. With respect to other poling techniques such as the UV poling,[16] thermal poling has significant advantages such as repeatability and much longer lifetime of the induced nonlinearity. Thermal poling involves applying to the glass a strong electric field, on the order of a few MV/m, at elevated temperatures, typically ~>250 °C, for ~10–15 minutes. This process induces a permanent second-order nonlinearity located in the first tens of microns below the anode surface of the poled glass. The nonlinearity is not uniform as a function of depth below this surface.

The main mechanism believed to be responsible for the second-order optical susceptibility, $\chi^{(2)}$, in thermally poled silica is the dc rectification of the third-order optical susceptibility of the glass, $\chi^{(3)}$. During poling, a space charge distribution develops near the poling anode, which creates a permanent dc electric field E. This built-in dc field rectifies the third-order susceptibility $\chi^{(3)}$ and produces a $\chi^{(2)}$ proportional to $\chi^{(3)}E$. Therefore, for poled silica, various nonlinear constants can be related to the built-in dc field as:[9]

$$d_{33} = 3d_{31} = \frac{\chi^{(2)}}{2} = \frac{3}{2} \cdot \chi^{(3)} \cdot E \qquad (10)$$

All the other nonzero elements of the nonlinear tensor in poled silica can be related to either d_{33} or d_{31}, with known proportionality constants.[9] In terms of SHG efficiency, a pure TM polarized fundamental wave generates the strongest SH (per unit thickness of poled silica), since the interaction of the fundamental and SH fields occur in this case through d_{33}, the strongest non-zero element of the nonlinear tensor in poled silica. A pure TE wave, on the other hand, interacts with its SH field through the weaker d_{31} coefficient (Eq. (10)). Furthermore, it is interesting to realize that for pure TM or pure TE polarized fundamental waves, the generated SH field will always be TM polarized. Only the co-existence of TM and TE polarizations in the fundamental wave allows the generation of TE polarized SH power from poled silica samples.

3.2.4.2 RECOVERED NONLINEARITY PROFILE OF POLED SILICA SAMPLES

The three IFT techniques described above were verified experimentally by testing each of them with the same two nonlinear samples. The samples were wafers of Infrasil 25x25x1 mm that were thermally poled under nominally identical, standard conditions, namely by placing each sample between silicon electrodes, heating the sample to ~270°C, then applying 5 kV across the electrodes for 15 min. At this point, the sample was cooled to room temperature and the voltage was turned off. The two samples were poled in this fashion one after the other. After thermal poling, sample B was ground and polished on its cathode side down to a thickness $L_B \approx 100$ μm. The purpose of this thinning step was to reduce the spacing between the two nonlinear regions in sandwich S2, and thus to reduce the frequency of oscillations at high angles in the MF curve of S2, which made its measurement easier.

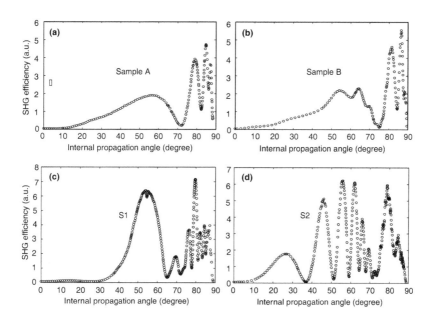

Fig. 10. (a), (b), (c), (d) Experimentally measured MF curves for sample A, sample B, S1 and S2 configurations.

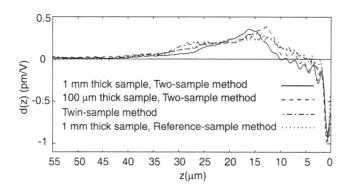

Fig. 11. Result of the recovered nonlinearity profile for poled silica samples using all three IFT techniques.

The experimental setup used to conduct these measurements is described in Appendix C (see Fig. C4). As illustrated in Fig. 1(b), in each measurement an Infrasil half-cylinder was clamped on the input surface of the sample under test to eliminate loss of fundamental power due to Fresnel reflection, and a second half-cylinder was placed against the output surface of the sample to eliminate TIR at that surface at high incidence angles and thus be able to measure MF curves up to very large angles.[5] The measured input fundamental peak power and output SH peak power were used to compute the SHG efficiency, which was plotted against internal propagation angle to obtain a MF curve.

Although for some of the IFT techniques only one MF curve needs to be measured, for completeness and cross-checks we measured the MF curve of four samples, namely sample A, sample B, sandwich S1, and sandwich S2. The four measured MF curves are plotted in Fig. 10. As expected, Maker-fringe curves MF_A and MF_B are very similar, since samples A and B are nominally identical and were poled under nominally identical conditions. The nonlinearity strengths of unpolished sample A (Fig. 10(a)) and polished sample B (Fig. 10(b)) are comparable, which suggests that there is no significant induced nonlinearity in the bulk of the material and in the vicinity of the cathode surface. MF_{S2} oscillates more prominently, and oscillations begin at smaller angles, because the two nonlinear regions are further apart in this sandwich than in sandwich S1 ($L \approx 140$ μm vs. ~40 μm). For each MF curve, prior to processing the experimental data points (which typically numbered ~300) were interpolated to generate additional points and improve the spatial resolution in the recovered profiles.

The profiles recovered using the two-sample technique are plotted in Fig. 11 (solid and dashed curves). The two profiles are very similar in shape and magnitude, which is expected since they were poled under identical conditions. Since samples A and B have similar profiles, one can also retrieve these two profiles by assuming that they are identical and applying the twin-sample method, for example, to MF_{S1}. The profile recovered by this method is the dot-dashed curve in Fig. 11. Finally, to apply the reference-sample technique, sample A was assumed to be the unknown sample and sample B the reference sample. The profile of sample B was selected as the profile measured by the two-sample technique (dashed curve in Fig. 11). The profile of sample A retrieved using the reference-sample technique is shown in Fig. 11 as the dotted curve. When this work was done in 2003, these results were quite exciting because it was the first time that the nonlinearity depth profile of a thermally poled silica sample was derived unambiguously. As expected, all recovered profiles are very similar. They share important features that were not recognized before these techniques were developed: (1) the nonlinear coefficient peaks about 1μm below the anode surface; (2) its magnitude is ~0.8-0.9 pm/V; (3) the nonlinear coefficient changes sign about 5 μm below the surface; and (4) the nonlinear region extends ~40 μm below the anode surface. The similarity between all these inferred profiles (even using different techniques) establishes that the three techniques are consistent, and it gives credibility to our results and to all three techniques. The small differences between the recovered profiles of sample A and B may partly be due to slight variations in the poling conditions. The sign reversal is also consistent with earlier reports from other research groups, both theoretical and experimental.[22-25]

It should be noted that neither the two-sample[3] nor the twin-sample technique[2] provides the overall sign of the recovered nonlinearity profile. The reference-sample technique,[4] on the other hand, does unambiguously retrieve this sign, provided the reference sample has a known sign. In most applications, this is a minor concern because knowledge of the absolute sign is not critical. Furthermore, the sign of the nonlinear crystal can be determined by independent means. For instance, in the present case of thermally poled silica, since the induced nonlinearity is mainly due to the dc rectification of the third-order susceptibility of the glass (Eq. (10)), at a given depth inside the nonlinear sample, the slope of the profile should give the polarity of the space charge at that depth. Independent measurements on samples poled under conditions similar to ours showed that the poled region has a negative charge ~5 μm beneath the anode surface, followed by a positively charged layer at ~10 μm, and finally a second layer of negative charge at ~30 μm.[19] This data enabled us to determine unambiguously the sign of the recovered profile, as shown in Fig. 11: the slope of the profile is first negative, then positive, and finally negative. This sequence agrees well with Ref. 19 in terms of both the number of space charge regions and their approximate depths. Another indication that the profiles of Fig. 11 have the correct sign can be obtained by integrating the recovered nonlinearity profile for along z, which gives the voltage drop across the nonlinear region. This integrated voltage comes out to be ~5.8 kV for the average of the profiles retrieved for the 1mm thick sample. As expected, this voltage has the same sign and roughly the same magnitude as the 5 kV applied during poling, which further supports the accuracy of the inferred profiles.

Even though all IFT techniques give very similar profiles, the profiles obtained by the two-sample technique are probably the most accurate because this method does not assume that the two profiles are identical. In contrast, the twin-sample technique assumes that sample A and sample B are identical. This assumption is validated by the fact that the two samples were poled under nominally identical conditions. However, the individual MF curves are very similar, but not identical (see Figs. 10(a) and 10(b)). This observation hints that the profiles differ a little, as is apparent in the two profiles retrieved by the two-sample technique shown in Fig. 11. The twin-sample technique is therefore expected to introduce some error in the nonlinearity profile it provides. It would be expected that it generates a profile that is some average of the actual profiles of samples A and B, which is indeed the case (Fig. 11). This limitation of the twin-sample technique can be reduced by cutting an unknown sample in two pieces and using these two pieces as samples A and B. Then the remaining source of error is possible non-uniformity in the nonlinearity profile across the face of two pieces, to which the twin-sample technique is more susceptible than the two-sample technique.

The reference-sample technique also relies on an additional piece of information, namely the profile of the reference sample. Consequently, any error made during the characterization of the reference profile is transferred to the profile of the unknown sample that was characterized using the reference-sample technique. However, this is not a fundamental limitation; it can be eliminated, for example, by using a thin film of known nonlinear material, such as $LiNbO_3$ or KDP, as the reference sample. The reference-sample profile is then a perfect rectangular function, and no error is introduced. This option makes the reference-sample technique potentially the most attractive and convenient of the three techniques, especially given its other practical benefits of higher speed, ease of coding, and reduced number of MF measurements.

3.2.5 FURTHER DISCUSSIONS ON THE ANALYTICAL RECOVERY TECHNIQUES

Application of other signal processing tools to the techniques described in this chapter opens a door for improvements of the recovery under different conditions. However, because the MF measurement system is not a "linear" system, one should, in general, be cautious. To illustrate this, let us assume that MF technique (MFT) is applied to nonlinear profiles $d_1(z)$ and $d_2(z)$, i.e., $d_1(z) \xrightarrow{\quad MFT \quad} |D_1(f)|$ and $d_1(z) \xrightarrow{\quad MFT \quad} |D_2(f)|$. For a linear combination of $d_1(z)$ and $d_2(z)$, the response of MFT would be $k_1 d_1(z) + k_2 d_2(z) \xrightarrow{\quad MFT \quad} |k_1 D_1(f) + k_2 D_1(f)|$, where k_1 and k_2 are arbitrary constants. Since, in general, $k_1|D_1(f)| + k_2|D_1(f)| \neq |k_1 D_1(f) + k_2 D_1(f)|$, an MF measurement is a nonlinear system. This nonlinearity is due simply to the fact that an MF experiment provides the *absolute* value of the FT of the nonlinearity profile. Therefore, special attention must be paid whenever a tool in signal processing is applied to improve the results of this paper. For instance, because of this nonlinearity, the application of the concept of "impulse response" to the MFT to improve the resolution would be meaningless.

Another issue is that $D(f = 0) = |D(0)| exp(j\phi(0)) = \int d(z) \cdot dz$, i.e., the integral of $d(z)$ across the entire wafer is the only determining factor for $D(0)$. This single data point $(f = 0)$ is important in a number of ways, especially for poled nonlinear samples. First, it can be used to check the convergence of the PG algorithm or in general, any algorithm used to extrapolate the measured FT spectrum into the low-frequency region ($[-f_{min}, f_{min}]$). By a direct integration of Eq. (10), one can prove that $|D(0)| = \left| \int d(z) \cdot dz \right| \leq \frac{3}{2} \cdot \chi^{(3)} \cdot V_p$, where V_p is the poling voltage and $\chi^{(3)}$ is the third-order optical susceptibility of the bulk material, it follows that the value of $|D(0)|$ obtained with the PG extrapolation algorithm should satisfy this inequality. Second, the value of $|D(0)|$ provides a means of checking the result of the recovery of $d(z)$ by ensuring that $\left| \int d(z) \cdot dz \right| = |D(0)|$ is satisfied. Finally, since $\int d(z) \cdot dz > 0$ implies $\phi(0) = 0$ and $\int d(z) \cdot dz < 0$ implies $\phi(0) = \pi$, for poled glasses, knowing the polarity of the voltage applied during poling means at the same time knowing whether $\phi(0)$ is equal to 0 or π, which might then be used either to check the recovered phase or to correct it.

Another important point to consider is that $d_{max} \leq \int_{-\infty}^{\infty} |D(f)| df$, which implies that a classical MF measurement of a nonlinear sample provides a simple upper bound value of the nonlinear coefficient of the sample.

Application of other signal processing tools to further improve the quality, ease and speed of the recovery process are left for future work.

3.3 ITERATIVE PROCESSING OF SECOND-ORDER OPTICAL NONLINEARITY DEPTH PROFILES

So far, we have demonstrated three analytical IFT techniques, where two nonlinear samples, either identical or different, are pressed against each other and the MF curve of this sandwich is measured. As a result of interference between the fundamental and SH signals within the two samples, the MF curve now includes information not only about the magnitude but also the phase of the FT. With analytical processing of this MF curve, it is now possible to recover the complete complex FT (amplitude and phase), which is then inverted to retrieve the profile $d(z)$ of the two samples unambiguously.

In this second part of Chapter 3, we present a much simpler technique to uniquely recover a nonlinearity profile from the classical MF measurement of a *single* sample instead of sandwich structures. This technique makes use of the iterative error reduction algorithms, introduced in Chapter 2 such as the Fienup algorithm[27] or the Gerchberg-Saxton algorithm[28]. We show that for a broad range of profiles, this family of algorithms enables the accurate recovery of the missing FT phase and thus, of the nonlinearity profile. This approach constitutes a substantial improvement over the analytical techniques discussed in the previous section, because of the simplicity of both the measurement and the computer code. The error in the recovered profile is also reduced. Furthermore, we show that this same iterative technique can be used to improve the accuracy of the profiles retrieved by any of the analytical techniques of Section 3.2.

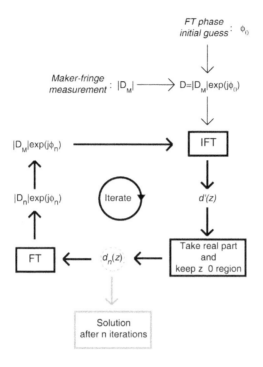

FT phase initial guess: ϕ_0

Maker-fringe measurement: $|D_M|$ $\longrightarrow$ $D = |D_M| \exp(j\phi_0)$

$|D_M| \exp(j\phi_n)$ $\longrightarrow$ IFT

$|D_n| \exp(j\phi_n)$ Iterate $d'(z)$

FT $\longleftarrow$ $d_n(z)$ $\longleftarrow$ Take real part and keep $z \geq 0$ region

Solution after n iterations

Fig. 12. Flow chart of the iterative error-reduction algorithm applied to recover nonlinearity profile of thin films.

3.3.1 ITERATIVE PROCESSING OF $d(z)$ USING ERROR-REDUCTION ALGORITHMS

The Fienup algorithm[27] and the Gerchberg-Saxton algorithm[28] are two of several iterative error-reduction algorithms that have been proposed to recover a function from partial information about this function in the space (or time) and/or Fourier domain. As discussed in Chapter 2, this family of algorithms uses the known (i.e., measured) FT magnitude of some unknown function $f(t)$, together with known properties of this function, such as being real or causal, and iteratively corrects an initial guess for $f(t)$. In the context of the present work, we use the iterative error-reduction algorithm to recover the nonlinearity spatial profile $d(z)$ of a thin (up to hundreds of microns) nonlinear sample from the measured MF curve of this sample. Note that without loss of generality, we can assume that $d(z)$ is a real and causal function, i.e., $d(z) = 0$ for $z < 0$, where $z = 0$ defines the edge of the wafer. As has been proved in the previous sections, the MF measurement of a single sample provides the magnitude of the spectrum $|D_M(f)|$ of the FT of $d(z)$, where f is the spatial frequency,[1] but it does not provide the phase spectrum $\phi(f)$ of this FT. The role of the iterative error-reduction algorithm, e.g., the Fienup algorithm, is to recover this missing FT phase. A basic flow chart of the iterative error-reduction algorithm applied to recover nonlinearity profile of thin films is shown in Fig. 12. To start, one makes an initial guess, $\phi_0(f)$, for the unknown FT phase (Fig. 12). We have found empirically that this initial guess does not strongly impact the convergence of the algorithm, so for convenience it can simply be $\phi_0(f) = 0$. As illustrated in Fig. 12, the first step in the algorithm is to calculate numerically the IFT of the complex quantity $|D_M(f)|\exp(j\phi_0(f))$. The second step is to take the real part of this IFT and retain only the $z \geq 0$ region, which gives a function $d_1(z)$ that constitutes a first estimate of the nonlinearity profile. The third and final step is to compute the FT of this profile, $|D_1(f)|\exp(j\phi_1(f))$. The phase $\phi_1(f)$ of this FT provides a new estimate for the missing FT phase $\phi(f)$. At this point, the FT of $d(z)$ has a known (measured) amplitude $|D_M(f)|$ and a best-estimate (calculated) phase $\phi_1(f)$. The previous three-step cycle is then repeated, using $\phi_1(f)$ instead of $\phi_0(f)$ as the new FT phase, which yields a second estimate $d_2(z)$ for the profile and a second estimate of the FT phase $\phi_2(f)$. This process is iterated n times until convergence is achieved, i.e., until the average difference between the profiles $d_{n-1}(z)$ and $d_n(z)$ obtained during two consecutive cycles is less than a preset value, for example 0.1%. The algorithm has reconstructed a more accurate spectrum $\phi_n(f)$ than the initial guess for the originally unknown FT phase.

As illustrated in Chapter 2, the Fienup algorithm always converges to *the* minimum-phase function whose FT magnitude is $|D_M(f)|$. Since this solution is unique, if we knew *a priori* that the profile to be reconstructed was an MPF (or close to being one), then we would be certain that the solution provided by the Fienup algorithm is the correct profile. The nonlinearity profile of poled silica, as discussed in Section 3.2.4.2, typically exhibits a sharp dominant peak just below the sample's anodic surface, which is related mostly to the injection of charges during the poling process from the anodic surface. Actually, all the functions shown in Fig. 1 of Chapter 2, which were accurately recovered from their FT magnitudes *alone*, were physically possible nonlinearity profiles for poled glasses or for thin sputtered films. This suggests that the iterative algorithm of Fig. 12 should work well for poled silica or for thin sputtered films as will be demonstrated in the next section. Furthermore, as illustrated in Fig. 4 of Chapter 2, the fact that increasing the magnitude of a function at the origin makes it close to being an MPF opens the possibility of recovering uniquely *any* nonlinearity profile by depositing on it a stronger and very thin nonlinear material, such as $LiNbO_3$. The film should be preferably thin because it is easier both to deposit and to measure its MF curve.

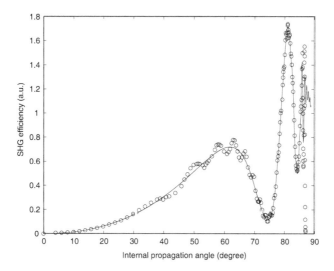

Fig. 13. Measured MF curve of the poled sample (circles) compared with the theoretically computed MF curve of the processed nonlinearity profile (solid curve).

It is important to point out two minor limitations of this processing technique. First, it cannot recover the exact location of the profile within the sample, i.e., how deeply $d(z)$ is buried below the surface of sample. Second, it cannot determine unequivocally the sign of the nonlinearity profile. Consequently, if $d_n(z)$ is the solution provided by the Fienup algorithm for a given nonlinear sample, then all $\pm d_n(z-z_0)$ functions are also solutions. However, in many cases, these limitations are fairly inconsequential; being able to determine the shape of a nonlinearity profile is much more important than determining its sign or exact location. Furthermore, if necessary, both the sign and location of $d(z)$ can be determined by other means, for example by using the reference-sample IFT technique.[4]

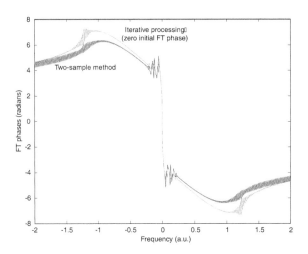

Fig. 14. Recovered FT phases with the two-sample technique and with the Fienup algorithm, assuming zero initial FT phase.

3.3.2 APPLICATION TO EXPERIMENTAL POLED SILICA SAMPLES

To verify the applicability of this processing technique to practical nonlinear materials, we tested it on a wafer of poled silica. The sample, a 25x25x0.15 mm wafer of fused silica (Infrasil), was thermally poled in air at 270 °C and ~4.8 kV for 15 min. In a first step, the MF spectrum of this sample was measured and the Fienup algorithm was applied to it, assuming zero initial FT phase, to recover a first nonlinearity profile. In a second step, the same sample was characterized by the two-sample IFT technique,[3] which produced a second, absolute nonlinearity profile. The hope was, of course, that the two profiles were the same. The setup used for these MF measurements has already been discussed earlier.

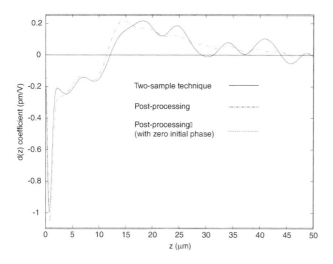

Fig. 15. Nonlinearity profiles recovered with the two-sample technique and with the Fienup algorithm.

Figure 13 shows the measured MF spectrum (open circles), which again is proportional to the square of the FT amplitude, $\left|D_M(f)\right|^2$, of $d(z)$. The maximum achieved internal propagation angle (θ_{max}) in this measurement is ~87°. However a large θ_{max} of this sort is not necessary, e.g., even $\theta_{max} \sim 78°$ is shown to supply adequate information for a fairly accurate recovery of the nonlinearity profile.[1] The FT phase and the profile recovered from this spectrum using the Fienup algorithm are plotted in Fig. 14 and Fig. 15, respectively. For comparison, on the same two figures, we also plotted the FT phase and the profile, respectively, recovered by the two-sample IFT technique.[3] The profiles retrieved by the Fienup algorithm and by the two-sample IFT technique are in excellent agreement: both exhibit a sharp nonlinearity coefficient peak of magnitude $d_{33} \approx 1$ pm/V just below the surface of the sample, a sign reversal at a depth of about 12 μm, and a wider positive nonlinear region extending to a depth of about 45 μm. These observations are in accord with profiles obtained using other IFT techniques in similar poled samples.[1-5] The FT phase spectra recovered by these two very different techniques (Fig. 14) are also in very good agreement. These excellent agreements lend support to both our iterative processing technique and the two-sample technique.

So far, we have always assumed a zero initial FT phase $\phi_0(f) = 0$ when using our processing algorithm. Now that we have access to the FT phase recovered by the two-sample technique (see Fig. 14), we can run our iterative processing algorithm using this spectrum instead of zero, as a better initial guess for this FT phase. This operation is equivalent to using our algorithm to post-process the FT phase recovered by the IFT technique, with the hope to obtain an even more accurate nonlinearity profile. The profile obtained by this post-processing technique after 100 iterations is shown as the dot-dashed curve in Fig. 15. A comparison to the profile obtained with the two-sample IFT technique (Fig. 15, solid curve) shows that while post-processing did not modify the overall profile shape, it significantly smoothed out the artificial oscillations introduced by the analytical IFT technique. The post-processed profile of the two-sample technique (dot-dashed curve) and the profile obtained with the Fienup algorithm assuming zero initial phase (dotted curve) are very close: the average difference between them is only 0.14%, which clearly demonstrates the validity of both approaches. The similarity between the profiles before and after post-processing confirms that the IFT technique came very close to recovering the actual profile. It also demonstrates the usefulness of our processing algorithm in another application, namely post-processing a profile obtained by an IFT technique. To better illustrate the beauty of this post-processing technique, we show in Fig. 13 the MF spectrum of the post-processed nonlinearity profile, calculated numerically (solid curve). There is very good agreement between this theoretical curve and the measured MF data (open circles).

We have tested this post-processing technique with the other two IFT techniques[2,4] and found that in all cases, post-processing significantly attenuates unphysical oscillations in the profile. The iterative post-processing technique is consequently a powerful tool to improve the accuracy of nonlinearity profiles recovered by an IFT technique. This processing step is also relatively fast: on a 500-MHz computer, 100 iterations typically take only a few seconds. Note also that the Fienup loop converges much faster if the thickness W of the nonlinear region is known. By knowing this thickness at the outset, $d(z)$ can be set to 0 not only over the $z < 0$ space but also for $z >$

W, which restricts the range of z values over which $d(z)$ is unknown. Thus, the iterative loop does not need to recover as many discrete values of $d(z)$ and converges faster.

3.4 SUMMARY

In this chapter, analytical and iterative techniques to uniquely recover the second-order nonlinearity depth profile of thin films are discussed and illustrated with numerical and experimental results. In the first half of Chapter 3, the fundamental limitation of the classical MF technique has been overcome by measuring the MF curve generated by the interference of two samples, instead of a single sample. This enabled us to retrieve the FT phase of $d(z)$ that could not be measured with the classical MF technique, which then led to the unique recovery of $d(z)$ profile of nonlinear films (e.g., poled silica films) by a simple IFT operation. For the most general case (the two-sample technique), we have shown that the two samples in our technique can be arbitrarily different, which then requires two MF measurements, i.e., S1 and S2 configurations. However, when the two samples are identical (the twin-sample technique) or one of them is an already known reference sample (the reference-sample technique), the nonlinearity profile can be characterized with a single MF measurement. The theory revealed that these two simpler approaches are actually special cases of the general theory of the two-sample technique. All significant details of these three analytical IFT techniques[2-4], including the frequency extrapolation algorithm used to complete the measured MF curves and the recovery algorithm of each technique, have been described.

The error analysis, conducted numerically, shows that all three of the analytical IFT techniques are quite robust to various measurement errors and/or limitations (e.g., limited θ_{max}) in terms of reliable recovery the $d(z)$ profile. In particular, the average error in the recovered profile is shown to be about 4 times smaller than the mean error in the measured MF curve. We have also shown that depending on the level of error present in the measurement system, there exists an optimum maximum measured angle, θ_{max}, which gives the best recovery (e.g., $\theta_{max} = 82°$ for one particular numerical simulation).

Verification of the theory for all three methods is also shown with thermally poled silica samples: the nonlinear coefficient peaks at ~1μm below the anode surface with a magnitude of ~0.9 pm/V, and extends ~40 μm below the anode surface with a sign change at 5-10 μm depth.

In the second half of Chapter 3, we have shown through numerical simulations and experimental data that a fast and simple iterative error-reduction loop known as the Fienup algorithm can be used to process the measured Maker fringe curve of a *single* nonlinear sample to accurately retrieve both the shape and the magnitude of the sample's nonlinearity profile. The Fienup algorithm works extremely well with profiles that are minimum-phase functions: for common minimum-phase functions, such as a buried Gaussian or an exponential, the average error is less than 0.004% after 100 iterations. We also demonstrated that the algorithm converges to a solution very close to the exact profile not only for minimum-phase functions but also for noisy minimum-phase functions and more generally for any profile that exhibits a dominant peak close to the origin, which covers a very wide range of practical nonlinearity profiles. This is true in particular of a rectangular profile, which is not a true minimum-phase function but does exhibit a dominant peak. The Fienup algorithm is therefore predicted to work well (average error of 0.008%) for deposited films of nonlinear crystals (e.g., $LiNbO_3$) or nonlinear organic materials. This is also true of profiles with two comparable peaks (average error of 0.1%) and even three-peak functions (error of a few %). Furthermore, the same iterative algorithm can be applied to the nonlinear profile obtained by an IFT technique to improve the profile accuracy, in particular to remove unphysical oscillations introduced by the IFT technique data processing algorithm. The validity of these conclusions was verified experimentally with a nonlinear sample of poled silica. The profile recovered from the measured MF curve of this sample using the Fienup algorithm was found to be in very good agreement with the profile of the same sample measured using an analytical IFT technique[3].

REFERENCES

1. A. Ozcan, M. J. F. Digonnet, G. S. Kino, "Detailed analysis of inverse Fourier transform techniques to uniquely infer second-order nonlinearity profile of thin films," J. Appl. Phys. 97, 013502 1 (2005)

2. A. Ozcan, M. J. F. Digonnet, G. S. Kino, "Inverse Fourier transform technique to determine second-order optical nonlinearity spatial profiles," Appl. Phys. Lett. 82, 1362 (2003)

3. A. Ozcan, M. J. F. Digonnet, G. S. Kino, "Improved technique to determine second-order optical nonlinearity profiles using two different samples," Appl. Phys. Lett. 84, 681 (2004)

4. A. Ozcan, M. J. F. Digonnet, and G. S. Kino, "Simplified inverse Fourier transform technique to measure optical nonlinearity profiles using reference sample," Electron. Lett. 40, 551 (2004)

5. A. Ozcan, M. J. F. Digonnet, and G. S. Kino, "Cylinder-assisted Maker-fringe technique," Electron. Lett. 39, 1834 (2003)

6. A. Ozcan, M. J. F. Digonnet, and G. S. Kino, "Iterative processing of second-order optical nonlinearity depth profiles," Opt. Express 12, 3367 (2004)

7. P. D. Maker, R W. Terhune, M. Nisenhoff, and C. M. Savage, "Effects of dispersion and focusing on production of optical harmonics," Phys. Rev. Lett. 8, 21 (1962)

8. H. G. Chatellus, et al., "Nondestructive method for the characterization of the second-order nonlinear profile and charge distribution in thermally poled fused silica," Opt. Lett. 25, 1723 (2000)

9. A. C. Liu, "Poled silica: Material and device characterization," Ph.D. dissertation submitted to the Department of Electrical Engineering, Stanford University, Stanford, CA (1999)

10. A. Kudlinski, et al., "Complete characterization of the nonlinear spatial distribution induced in poled silica glass with a submicron resolution," Appl. Phys. Lett. 83, 3623 (2003)

11. A. L. C. Triques, et al., "Time evolution of depletion region in poled silica," Appl. Phys. Lett. 82, 2948 (2003)

12. A. Papoulis, "New algorithm in spectral analysis and band-limited extrapolation," IEEE Trans. Circuits, Syst. 22, 735 (1975)

13. R. W. Gerchberg, "Super-resolution through error energy reduction," Opt. Acta. 21, 709 (1974)

14. P. J. S. G. Ferreira, "Interpolation and the discrete Papoulis-Gerchberg algorithm," IEEE Trans. on Signal Processing 42, 2596 (1994)

15. R. A. Myers, N. Mukerjkee, and S. R. J. Brueck, "Large second-order nonlinearity in poled fused silica," Opt. Lett. 16, 1732 (1991)

16. Y. Quiquempois, P. Niay, M. Douay, and B. Poumellec, " Advances in poling and permanently induced phenomena in silica-based glasses," Current Opinion in Solid State & Materials Science 7, 89 (2003)

17. M. Mukherjee, R. A. Myers, and S. R. J. Brueck, "Dynamics of second-harmonic generation in fused silica," J. Opt. Soc. Am. B 11, 665 (1994)

18. H. Takabe, P. G. Kazansky, P.S. J. Russell, and K. Morinaga, "Effect of poling conditions on second-harmonic generation in fused silica," Opt. Lett. 21, 468 (1996)

19. P.G. Kazansky, A. R. Smith, P. S. J. Russell, G. M. Yang, G. M. Sessler, "Thermally poled silica glass: laser induced pressure pulse probe of charge distribution," Appl. Phys. Lett. 68, 269 (1996)

20. T. G. Alley, S. R. J. Brueck, and R. A. Myers, "Space charge dynamics in thermally poled fused silica," J. Non-Cryst. Solids 242, 165 (1998)

21. D. Faccio, V. Pruneri, and P. G. Kazanksy, "Dynamics of the second order nonlinearity in thermally poled silica glass," Appl. Phys. Lett. 79, 2687 (2001)

22. P. Thamboon and D. M. Krol, "Second-order optical nonlinearities in thermally poled phosphate glasses," J. Appl. Phys. 93, 32 (2003)

23. A. Le Calvez, E. Freysz, and A. Ducasse, "A model for second harmonic generation in poled glasses," Eur. Phys. J. D 1, 223 (1998)

24. H. G. de Chatellus and E. Freysz, "Static and dynamic profile of the electric field within the bulk of fused silica glass during and after thermal poling," Opt. Lett. 28, 1624 (2003)

25. A. Kudlinski, Y. Quiquempois, H. Zeghlache, and G. Martinelli, "Evidence of second-order nonlinear susceptibility sign reversal in thermally poled samples," Appl. Phys. Lett. 83, 3242 (2003)

26. A. L. C. Triques, C. M. B. Cordeiro, V. Balestrieri, B. Lesche, W. Margulis, and I. C. S Carvalho, "Depletion region in thermally poled fused silica," Appl. Phys. Lett. 76, 2496 (2000)

27. J. R. Fienup, "Reconstruction of an object from the modulus of its Fourier transform," Opt. Lett. 3, 27 (1978)

28. R. W. Gerchberg and W. O. Saxton, "Practical algorithm for the determination of phase from image and diffraction plane pictures," Optik 35, 237-246 (1972)

CHAPTER 4: CHARACTERIZATION AND OPTIMIZATION OF THERMALLY POLED GERMANOSILICATE GLASSES

This chapter describes the characterization and the optimization of the induced second-order optical nonlinearity profile in thermally poled germanosilicate glasses, using the iterative characterization technique discussed in Chapter 3. Specifically, we report measurements of the nonlinearity profile of thermally poled low-loss germanosilicate films deposited on fused-silica substrates by plasma-enhanced chemical vapor deposition (PECVD), of interest as potential electro-optic devices. After local optimization, we demonstrate a record peak nonlinear coefficient of ~1.6 pm/V, approximately twice as strong as the highest reliable value reported in thermally poled fused silica glass, a significant improvement that was qualitatively expected from the doping of Ge. Fabrication, refractive index and optical loss characterization of the reported germanosilicate films were carried out by Feridun Ay and Prof. Atilla Aydinli of Bilkent University, Ankara, Turkey. All the thermal poling of the grown thin films, characterization measurements, and the relevant data analysis together with the principles of the theory were primarily conducted by Aydogan Ozcan under the supervision of Gordon S. Kino and Michel J. F. Digonnet. Parts of this chapter have already been published in *Optics Express* Vol. 12, 4698, (2004).

4.1 INTRODUCTION

In this chapter, we report a poling study of germanosilicate films that makes significant progress towards achieving practical poled-glass electro-optic devices. First, the *peak* magnitude of the induced nonlinearity is improved from earlier results by roughly a factor of two (~1.6 pm/V).[1-6] Second, recovering a detailed map of the induced nonlinearity profile enabled us to optimize the overlap of the optical mode with the nonlinearity profile in integrated electro-optic modulators, which resulted in the highest reported *effective* nonlinearity in poled-glass based integrated devices (~0.32 pm/V). This work is the logical sequel of the powerful nonlinear material characterization tools introduced in Chapter 3.

The choice of germanosilicate glass was made for two reasons. First, since their propagation loss has been dramatically reduced,[7] germanosilicate films grown onto fused silica substrates are excellent waveguides with a refractive index close to that of silica, which makes them compatible with fiber-optic technology. Second, the addition of Ge to silica increases the refractive index of the glass, and thus its third-order optical susceptibility $\chi^{(3)}$, and since the nonlinear coefficient d_{33} of poled glass is proportional to $\chi^{(3)}$ it is expected that d_{33} will also be increased. Poled germanosilicate glass[6,8,9] is therefore a promising candidate for low-loss as-deposited integrated planar electro-optic devices. In this work, we used thermal poling instead of UV poling because the latter produces strong but short-lived nonlinear regions.[9] We confirm these expectations with experimental investigations, showing that the peak nonlinear coefficient of germanosilicate films with optimal Ge concentration, thickness, and poling time exhibit a record value of ~1.6 pm/V. Precise and unique characterization of the spatial profile of the nonlinear region, using the iterative processing technique developed in Chapter 3,[10] reveals interesting details regarding the physics of poling in these glasses, including the fact that the Ge-doped layer blocks diffusion of the positive ions from the anode surface during poling and that the space charge distribution inside the poled region exhibits a dipolar structure within the first micron below the anode surface, followed by a neutral region from ~1 μm to ~12 μm, which is followed by a weaker negatively charged region up to a total depth of ~16 μm. These findings are important, especially for optimizing the overlap of the optical mode of an electro-optic device utilizing poled germanosilicate films onto the induced nonlinear region.

4.2 GERMANOSILICATE GROWTH PROCESS

The germanosilicate films were deposited on square substrates of synthetic silica (Infrasil) 25 mm on the side and 150 μm thick, using plasma-enhanced chemical vapor deposition (PECVD) in a parallel-plate reactor (Plasmalab 8510C). The films were grown at 350 °C and at a pressure of 1 Torr, with an RF power of 10 W at 13.56 MHz applied to the plates. The diameter of the plates was 24 cm. The precursor gases were silane (2% SiH_4/N_2), germane (2% GeH_4/He), and nitrous oxide (N_2O). The flow rates of silane and nitrous oxide were kept constant at 180 and 225 sccm, respectively, while that of germane was set at a constant value between 0 and 90 sccm that was varied from run to run. The growth rate of the films was ~40 nm/min.

A major problem in the application of CVD-grown silicon-based layers in integrated optics is the incorporation of hydrogen in the form of N–H bonds into the film matrix.[11] Annealing is usually required to reduce the propagation loss of the optical waveguides that utilize these layers as the core. Instead, the samples were manufactured using a new recipe that has produced the lowest propagation loss of as-grown germanosilicate films reported to date.[7]

Table 1. Characteristics and poling time of germanosilicate films poled in air at ~5 kV and ~280 °C.

Sample #	Germane flow rate	Mole fraction of GeO_2 (%)	Refractive index at 1064nm	Thickness	Poling time	Peak d_{33} (pm/V)
1	0 sccm	0	1.469	4 µm	10 min	0.54
2	33 sccm	~20	1.497	4 µm	5 min	0.80
3	33 sccm	~20	1.497	4 µm	10 min	1.59
4	33 sccm	~20	1.497	4 µm	15 min	1.00
5	33 sccm	~20	1.497	2 µm	10 min	1.02
6	50 sccm	~30	1.514	4 µm	10 min	0.78
7	90 sccm	~56	1.553	4 µm	10 min	0.81

In order to study the effects of film composition, film thickness, and poling time on the nonlinearity profile and strength of poled germanosilicate films, seven germanosilicate films at four different germane flow rates (0, 33, 50, and 90 sccm) were grown. The characteristics of these films and the poling times are listed in Table 1. Mole fraction of GeO_2 of the grown films is estimated from the measured dispersion curves of the films, as listed in Table 1.[12] Based on previous measurements of similar samples,[7] the propagation loss of the as-grown waveguides was estimated to be less than 0.15 dB/cm at 1550 nm.

4.3. THERMAL POLING AND CHARACTERIZATION OF THE POLED FILMS

As-grown germanosilicate-Infrasil structures were thermally poled[13] using polished *n*-type silicon electrodes in air at ~5 kV and 280 °C, with the positive electrode facing the film. The nonlinearity spatial profile of each poled sample was measured using the Maker fringe-Fienup technique described in the second half of Chapter 3.[10,14,15] Because of the refractive index mismatch between the Infrasil substrate and the germanosilicate film, angle-dependent spurious reflections occurred at the film-cylinder and the film-substrate interfaces. Correction factors were thus applied to the measured MF curves to correct them for multiple reflections[16] and Fresnel reflection at both the fundamental and SH signal wavelengths. Furthermore, the sample grown at a 90-sccm germane flow rate, which physically looked brown, had higher loss, especially in the visible spectrum. The film's measured loss coefficients (~4 dB/cm at 1064 nm and ~710 dB/cm at 532 nm) were thus used to correct the measured MF curve for this poled sample. Finally, each of these corrected MF curves was processed using the iterative Fienup algorithm[17] described in Chapter 3 to uniquely recover the second-order optical nonlinearity profile of each poled sample. This approach was selected for its greater simplicity and speed over other inverse Fourier transform (FT) techniques, such as the two-sample technique[2]. Furthermore, for germanosilicate-Infrasil thin film structures, the MF curves of sandwich structures required by the inverse FT techniques would be more difficult to measure and calibrate, due to multiple reflections arising from the 4 interfaces with refractive index mismatch. Using the iterative Fienup algorithm avoids this complex situation, which also increases the accuracy of the recovery.

To identify the optimum poling time for these samples, we first poled samples #2, #3, and #4, all of which were grown at 33 sccm germane flow rate to a thickness of 4 µm, for 5, 10 and 15 minutes, respectively. The calibrated MF curves of these poled samples are shown in Figs. 1(a)-(c). The nonlinearity depth profile of each sample recovered from these curves is shown in Fig. 1(d). All three profiles exhibit similar features, namely a sharp peak centered about 0.5 µm below the anode, followed by a weak pedestal that is approximately constant to a depth of ~9–12 µm and gradually decreases to zero at a depth of 13–16 µm.

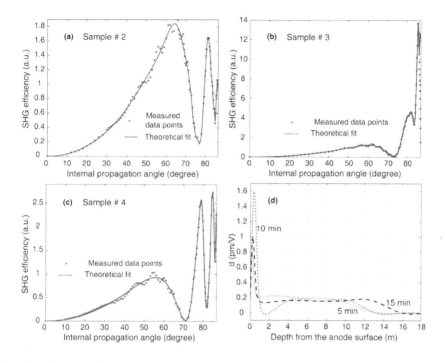

Fig. 1. Calibrated MF curves measured for (a) sample # 2, (b) sample # 3, and (c) sample # 4. The solid curves are the theoretical MF curves computed from the recovered $d_{33}(z)$ profiles. (d) The recovered optical nonlinearity depth profiles of sample # 2 (solid), # 3 (dotted) and # 4 (dashed).

This sequence of profiles reveals that the optimum poling time for these germanosilicate-Infrasil structures at an applied E-field of ~32.5 MV/m is about 10 min. The peak d_{33} coefficient obtained under these poling conditions is as high as ~1.6 pm/V. To our knowledge, this is the highest directly measured second-order nonlinear coefficient reported to date in thermally poled germanosilicate glass, and it is about twice as high as the highest reliable peak d_{33} value reported for thermally poled fused silica.[2] The other measured peak d_{33} coefficients for poling times of 5 and 15 min are ~0.8 pm/V and ~1.0 pm/V, respectively. Note that the entire nonlinearity peak is contained in the germanosilicate film, while most of the pedestal is in the silica substrate. Furthermore, as physically expected, due to the diffusion of positive ions, the depth of the pedestal gradually increases from ~9 μm to ~12 μm as the poling time is increased from 5 min to 15 min (see Fig. 1(d)).

As described in Chapter 3, the profiles recovered using the Fienup algorithm could be shifted in space from the actual profile, i.e., absolute recovery of the origin of the z axis is not possible with the iterative Fienup algorithm.[10] However, if the recovered profiles were shifted even slightly into the bulk of the sample, then this solution would imply an unpoled region a few micrometers deep under the anode electrode, with $d = 0$ pm/V. There is no physical evidence for such an unpoled region just under the anode electrode. For thermally poled materials, the observed trend is that the nonlinearity starts right at the anode surface, and extends into the substrate.[1,2,18-20] Therefore, the recovered nonlinearity profiles reported in Fig. 1 and in the rest of this chapter do not involve relative spatial shifts with respect to the anode surface.

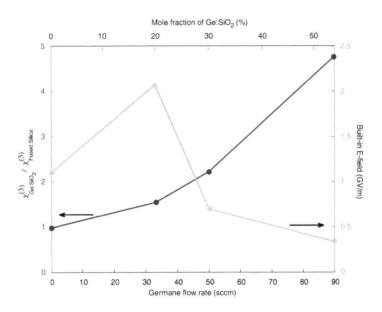

Fig. 2. Left axis: the ratio of the $\chi^{(3)}$ of the PECVD grown layer to the $\chi^{(3)}$ of fused silica; Right axis: maximum built-in E-field inferred from measurements in poled germanosilicate films.

As described in Chapter 3, we postulate that dc rectification mechanism is responsible for the nonlinearity of the present materials, and we attribute the observed increase in the peak d_{33} coefficient to the higher $\chi^{(3)}$ of germanosilicate. To validate this assumption, we used an empirical relationship[21] to predict the nonlinear refractive index of the germanosilicate films from their dispersion curves. The ratio of the third-order susceptibility of the PECVD grown layer, $\chi^{(3)}_{Ge:SiO_2}$, to the susceptibility of fused silica, $\chi^{(3)}_{FusedSilica}$, computed using the measured dispersion curves of the films grown at 0, 33, 50, and 90 sccm germane flow rates, is plotted in Fig. 2 as a function of the germane flow rate. This curve shows that (1) as expected physically, the $\chi^{(3)}$ of the 0-sccm germane flow rate film is very close to the $\chi^{(3)}$ of fused silica; (2) as the germane flow rate is increased, the $\chi^{(3)}$ of the germanosilicate film increases almost quadratically. Specifically, for sample #3 (flow rate of 33 sccm) $\chi^{(3)}_{Ge:SiO_2} \approx 1.54 \cdot \chi^{(3)}_{SiO_2}$. This enhancement factor contributes to ~1.54/2 ≈ 80% of the two-fold increase observed in the peak d_{33} coefficient of sample #3, which suggests that the remaining contribution should be due to a 30% increase in the built-in field in sample #3 compared to the built-in field of poled fused silica.[2]

The total depth of the induced nonlinear region (~13–16 µm) in Fig. 1(d) is significantly narrower than for bulk Infrasil samples thermally poled under similar conditions, for which the depth is typically ~40 µm.[2,10,22] Furthermore, unlike poled Infrasil samples, the $d_{33}(z)$ profile of the poled germanosilicate-Infrasil structures does not change sign. In our opinion, these differences occur because the germanosilicate film limits the diffusion of positive ions such as H_3O^+ from the anode surface into the sample, resulting in the formation of a narrower depletion region within the film itself. A similar blocking behavior in germanosilicate films, which also resulted in narrower nonlinear widths, has been previously reported.[8]

For comparison purposes, the theoretical MF curves computed from the inferred $d_{33}(z)$ profiles of Fig. 1(d) are also shown in Figs. 1(a)-(c) (solid curves). The excellent agreement between the computed and the measured MF curves for all three samples again confirms the high accuracy of the Maker fringe-Fienup technique and the validity of our results. Note that all of the measured MF curves exhibit faster small-amplitude oscillations superimposed on a much stronger but slower fundamental oscillation. This weak high frequency modulation is especially evident in the measured MF curve of sample #4 between internal propagation angles of 35° and 65° (see Fig. 1(c)). We believe that this fast oscillation is simply due to a much weaker nonlinearity induced at the cathode end of the poled samples, which has also been observed in other thermally-poled samples.[23-25] The period of this fast oscillation roughly matches the thickness of the poled samples (~150 μm), which supports our argument. Meanwhile, the theoretically computed MF curves (solid curves in Figs. 1(a)-(c)) corresponding to the recovered profiles do not show these fast oscillations but do show excellent agreement with the much stronger but slower oscillations in the measured MF curves. This expected result occurs because the Papoulis-Gerchberg algorithm (see Appendix B) was used to recover the full spatial FT spectrum from the measured MF curves. In this extrapolation algorithm, to speed up the convergence, the extent of the nonlinear region is limited to a depth of less than ~60 μm from the anode surface. Therefore, any nonlinear coefficient beyond this first 60 μm is neglected, including the weak nonlinearity at the cathode end. For practical device applications, e.g., electro-optic phase/amplitude modulators, this decision is quite reasonable since the most significant and useful part of the nonlinearity is confined to the first ~40 μm below the anode surface.[1,2,10] The fact that it is safe to neglect the nonlinearity after the first ~60 μm is also verified by that the reported theoretical MF curves all agree perfectly with the stronger slow oscillations of the measured MF curves (see Figs. 1(a)-(c)).

Assuming that dc rectification is the main mechanism responsible for the observed nonlinearity in poled silica samples, as discussed in Chapter 3, then the total voltage drop across the nonlinear region should be equal to the poling voltage.[22] To verify this assumption, we computed the integral along the depth z of each recovered nonlinearity profile of Fig. 1(d). The calculated voltages come out to be 4.77 kV, 4.77 kV and 5.21 kV for sample #2, #3 and #4, respectively. As expected, these values are close to the poling voltage (~5 kV), which lends further credence to the inferred profiles. As discussed in Chapter 3, the true sign of the profiles in Fig. 1(d) cannot be inferred by using the Fienup algorithm alone.[10] However, one way of resolving this sign ambiguity, as discussed in Chapter 3, is comparing the sign of the integral of the profile, with the sign of the poling voltage.[22] The fact that the integrated voltage drop across the recovered profiles has the same sign as the poling voltage (+5 kV) suggests that the inferred profiles as shown in Fig. 1(d) do have the correct sign (positive).

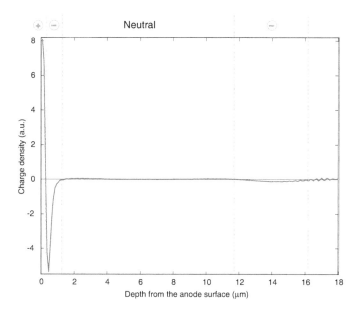

Fig. 3. Charge density of poled sample # 4, inferred by differentiating its recovered $d_{33}(z)$ profile shown in Fig. 1(d).

To provide further physical insight into the poling process for the germanosilicate-Infrasil structures, we calculated the charge density distribution frozen within the glass from the recovered nonlinearity profiles. Since the profile is proportional to the built-in E-field distribution, and since the distribution of space charge density in the glass is proportional to the derivative of the built-in E-field, the charge density can be obtained simply by taking the derivative of the measured profile. As an example, the charge density distribution of sample # 4 (Fig. 1(d)) recovered by this process is shown in Fig. 3. This distribution exhibits a dipolar structure within the first micron below the anode surface, followed by a neutral region from ~1.2 µm to ~11.5 µm, which in turn, is followed by a weaker negatively charged region extending to a depth of ~16.2 µm.

The charge distributions recovered for the other samples show very similar features, the main difference being minor variations in the locations of these regions. The integral of the recovered charge distribution shown in Fig. 3 yields a total charge of -8.53 10^{-3} C/m². We believe that the neutrality of the sample is preserved by an equal amount of positive alkali ion (e.g., Na⁺ or K⁺) charge that is spread throughout the remaining bulk of the Infrasil substrate. Because this charge density is spread over roughly 150 μm of glass, it is much lower, and thus it contributes to a bulk second-order nonlinearity that is too weak to be measured. Furthermore, we anticipate that the depth of the neutral region shown in Fig. 3 reflects the total diffusion depth of the positive ions injected from the anode surface, canceling out the negative sites left behind by alkali ions that have migrated towards the cathode.

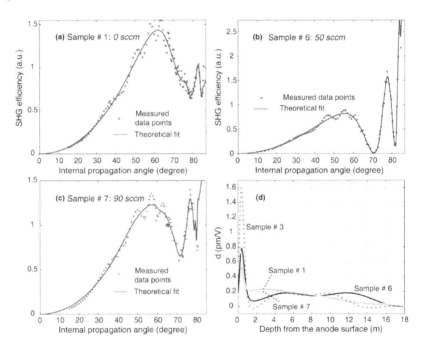

Fig. 4. Calibrated MF curves measured for (a) sample #1, (b) sample #6, and (c) sample #7. The solid curves in each figure are the theoretical MF curves computed from the recovered $d_{33}(z)$ profiles. (d) The recovered nonlinearity profiles of sample #1 (dot-dashed), #3 (dotted), #6 (dark solid), and #7 (light solid).

After optimizing the poling time, we investigated the effect of the germane flow rate on the induced nonlinearity profile. For this purpose, we poled samples #1, #3, #6, and #7, which all had 4-μm thick germanosilicate films but were grown with different flow rates, namely 0, 33, 50 and 90 sccm, respectively. The poling conditions for all four samples were identical, i.e., in air at ~5 kV and 280 °C, for 10 min. The calibrated measured MF curves for samples #1, #6, and #7 are shown in Figs. 4(a)-(c). The MF curve for sample #3 has already been shown in Fig. 1(b). The nonlinearity profiles recovered by applying the Fienup algorithm to these MF curves are shown in Fig. 4(d). The profiles exhibit the same characteristics as the previous samples (see Fig. 1(d)), i.e., a dominant peak buried ~0.5 µm beneath the anode surface, followed by an almost constant nonlinear region of same sign that gradually decreases to zero at a width of 13–16 µm. The peak d_{33} coefficients of samples #1, #6, and #7 were found to be 0.54, 0.78, and 0.81 pm/V, respectively. This investigation showed that the highest peak d_{33} coefficient (1.6 pm/V) was achieved for a germane flow of 33 sccm (sample #3).

Although a higher germane flow rate produces a higher Ge concentration and thus a higher $\chi^{(3)}$, as confirmed in Fig. 2, the fact that the peak d_{33} coefficient is maximum in the 33-sccm sample suggests that the built-in field drops at higher Ge flow rates. To illustrate this point, the maximum built-in E-field in poled germanosilicate films, calculated using the measured peak d_{33} value and the inferred $\chi^{(3)}$ value for each sample, is also plotted as a function of germane flow rate in Fig. 2. The results reveal that the highest built-in field is achieved for the 33-sccm sample (#3) and that for higher germane flow rates the built-in field steadily drops. We attribute these observations primarily to an increase in the film electrical conductivity as the Ge concentration is increased, as has been previously confirmed.[26] On the other hand, the built-in field of the 33-sccm sample is higher than that of the 0-sccm sample (pure SiO_2), although the latter has a lower electrical conductivity. Thus, there is an optimum electrical conductivity range for a given set of poling conditions. This hypothesis is supported by the fact that under similar poling conditions, Suprasil, which contains much less impurity than Infrasil and thus has a lower conductivity, develops a built-in field nearly one order of magnitude lower than Infrasil.[1,23] Furthermore, we should briefly note that our attempts to increase the built-in electric field by poling at higher poling voltages in excess of ~10 kV resulted in similar peak d_{33} values indicating that the breakdown electric field of the material is already reached. Actually this hypothesis is also verified by the fact that the poling current increased from sub nA to >100 nA when the poling voltage is increased from 5 kV to >10 kV, indicating an avalanche effect due to internal dielectric breakdown of the material.

It should be noted that the measured MF curves for samples #1 and #7 are quite similar, in both shape and strength (see Figs. 4(a) and 4(c)). This explains the similarity in the recovered nonlinearity profiles of these two samples, as can be seen in Fig. 4(d). However, the peak d_{33} coefficient is weaker for sample #1 (0.54 pm/V) than for sample #7 (0.81 pm/V). This difference originates from the second peak in the MF curves around an internal propagation angle of ~80°, which is stronger for sample #7 than for sample #1 (see Figs. 4(a) and 4(c)). At such high angles, the fundamental beam interacts primarily with the nonlinearity at the surface of the material because diffraction causes the power density of the fundamental beam to decrease in the substrate, which reduces the SH conversion efficiency in the deeper part of the nonlinearity profile. From the enhanced SHG efficiency observed near ~80°, we therefore expect a stronger nonlinearity close to the surface, as observed in the recovered profile of sample #7. Another way to look at the same phenomena is to consider that higher angles correspond to higher spatial Fourier transform frequencies, so the more slowly the high frequency components decay to zero, the more tightly confined the nonlinearity is. For example, in the limit where high frequency components never decay to zero, the profile is a delta function, i. e., all the nonlinearity is confined to the surface of the sample. This reasoning also explains the record peak nonlinearity observed in sample #3. In the measured MF curve of sample #3 (Fig. 1(b)), the SHG efficiency at high angles (e.g., 80° or higher) is about 5–7 times stronger than for all the other samples, an increase that is caused by the stronger nonlinearity present near the anode surface in sample #3. Overall, the fact that the strength of the nonlinearity peak close to the anode surface is mostly visible at higher angles establishes once again the importance of measuring MF curves up to high angles.[14]

Once again, for comparison purposes we also show the theoretical MF curves computed from the recovered profiles of Fig. 4(d) as solid curves in Figs. 4(a)-(c). The agreement between these theoretical and measured MF curves is again excellent, further supporting our results. The calculated total voltage drop across the nonlinear profiles of Fig. 4(d) is 4.92 kV, 5.58 kV, and 5.34 kV for samples #1, #6, and #7, respectively; all are in good agreement with the poling voltage (~5 kV).

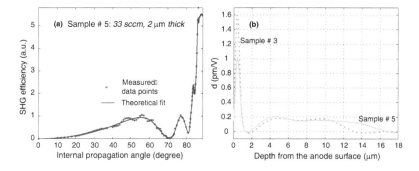

Fig. 5. Calibrated MF curve measured for (a) sample #5. The solid curves are the theoretical MF curves computed from the recovered $d_{33}(z)$ profiles. (b) The recovered optical nonlinearity depth profile of samples #3 (dashed) and #5 (solid).

Finally, we investigated the effect of film thickness on the induced nonlinearity profile. For this purpose, we poled sample #5, grown with a 33-sccm germane flow rate to a final thickness of 2 μm, in air at ~5 kV and 280 °C, for 10 min. Figure 5(a) shows the measured calibrated MF curve for sample #5, and Fig. 5(b) shows the nonlinearity profile recovered from this curve. For comparison purposes, the nonlinearity profile of sample #3, which was grown at the same flow rate and poled under identical conditions but is thicker (4 μm), is also shown in Fig. 5(b). Note again that the nonlinearity peak is entirely contained in the film and the pedestal in the substrate. The two samples (# 3 and # 5) have very similar profiles, which was expected, since they have the same material composition and were poled under the same conditions. However, the total depth of the nonlinearity is larger for sample #5 (~17 μm) than for sample #3 (~13 μm). This difference occurs primarily because the 2-μm thick germanosilicate film in sample #5 acts as a weaker barrier for ion diffusion process than the 4-μm film in sample #3. Furthermore, we believe that this charge spreading is at the origin of the weaker peak d_{33} coefficient in sample #5 (1.02 pm/V, vs. 1.6 pm/V in sample #3). Again, the theoretical MF curve computed from the recovered profile of Fig. 5(b) (solid curve in Fig. 5(a)) is in excellent agreement with the measured MF curve, and the calculated total voltage drop across the nonlinear profile of sample #5 (4.96 kV) agrees very well with the poling voltage (~5 kV).

4.4   CONCLUSIONS

We have reported measurements of the nonlinearity spatial profile of thermally poled germanosilicate films deposited on fused-silica substrates by PECVD. These films are particularly interesting: they exhibit a low propagation loss; and they were expected to have a stronger nonlinearity than poled undoped silica due to the presence of Ge, which increases the third-order susceptibility of the glass. Inferred profiles confirm these predictions. They all exhibit a sharp peak ~0.5 μm beneath the anode surface, followed by a weaker pedestal of roughly constant amplitude and same sign down to a depth of 13–16 μm. These profiles are shallower and do not exhibit the sign reversal typical of poled undoped silica, which suggests that during poling, the germanosilicate film significantly slows down the injection of positive ions from the anode surface into the structure. After optimizing the germane flow rate during deposition, the film thickness, and the poling time for maximum peak nonlinearity, we demonstrated a record peak nonlinear coefficient of ~1.6 pm/V, approximately twice as strong as the highest reliable value reported to date in a thermally poled fused silica glass. These findings are significant for the design of electro-optic devices using thermally poled germanosilicate thin films, especially for optimization of the overlap of the optical mode and the nonlinear region of the device.

REFERENCES

1. Y. Quiquempois, P. Niay, M. Douay, and B. Poumellec, " Advances in poling and permanently induced phenomena in silica-based glasses," Current Opinion in Solid State & Materials Science 7, 89 (2003)

2. A. Ozcan, M. J. F. Digonnet, and G. S. Kino, "Improved technique to determine second-order optical nonlinearity profiles using two different samples," Appl. Phys. Lett. 84, 681 (2004)

3. A. C. Liu, M. J. F. Digonnet, and G. S. Kino, "Electro-optic phase modulation in silica channel waveguide," Opt. Lett. 19, 466 (1994)

4. T. Fujiwara, D. Wong, and S. Fleming, "Large electrooptic modulation in a thermally-poled germanosilicate fiber," IEEE Photon. Tech. Lett. 10, 1177 (1995)

5. X. C. Long and S. R. J. Brueck, "Large-signal phase retardation with a poled electrooptic fiber," IEEE Photon. Tech. Lett. 9, 767 (1997)

6. Y. Ren, C. J. Marckmann, J. Arentoft, and M. Kristensen, "Thermally poled channel waveguides with polarization-independent electrooptic effect," IEEE Photon. Tech. Lett. 14, 639 (2002)

7. F. Ay, A. Aydinli, and S. Agan "Low-loss as-grown germanosilicate layers for optical waveguides," Appl Phys. Lett. 83, 4743 (2003)

8. D. Faccio, A. Busacca, D. W. J. Harwood, G. Bonfrate, V. Pruneri, and P. G. Kazansky, "Effect of core-cladding interface on thermal poling of germanosilicate optical waveguides," Opt. Comm. 196, 187 (2001)

9. J. Khaled, T. Fujiwara, M. Ohama, and A. J. Ikushima, "Generation of second harmonics in Ge-doped SiO_2 thin films by ultraviolet irradiation under poling electric field," J. Appl. Phys. 87, 2137 (2000)

10. A. Ozcan, M. J. F. Digonnet, and G. S. Kino, "Iterative processing of second-order optical nonlinearity depth profiles," Opt. Express 12, 3367 (2004), http://www.opticsexpress.org/abstract.cfm?URI=OPEX-12-15-3367

11. F. Ay, and A. Aydinli, "Comparative investigation of hydrogen bonding in silicon based PECVD grown dielectrics for optical waveguides," Opt. Mat. 26, 33 (2004)

12. A. S. Huang, Y. Arie, C. C. Neil, and J. M. Hammer, "Study of refractive index of $GeO_2:SiO_2$ mixtures using deposited-thin-film optical waveguides," Appl. Opt. 24, 4404 (1985)

13. R. A. Myers, N. Mukerjkee, and S. R. J. Brueck, "Large second-order nonlinearity in poled fused silica," Opt. Lett. 16, 1732 (1991)

14. A. Ozcan, M. J. F. Digonnet, and G. S. Kino, "Cylinder-assisted Maker-fringe technique," Electron. Lett. 39, 1834 (2003)

15. P. D. Maker, R. W. Terhune, M. Nisenhoff, and C. M. Savage, "Effects of dispersion and focusing on production of optical harmonics," Phys. Rev. Lett. 8, 21 (1962)

16. J. Jerphagnon, and S. K. Kurtz, "Maker fringes: a detailed comparison of theory and experiment for isotropic and uniaxial crystals," J. Appl. Phys. 41, 1667 (1970)

17. J. R. Fienup, "Reconstruction of an object from the modulus of its Fourier transform," Opt. Lett. 3, 27 (1978)

18. T. G. Alley, S. R. J. Brueck, and R. A. Myers, "Space charge dynamics in thermally poled fused silica," J. Non-Cryst. Solids 242, 165 (1998)

19. A. C. Liu, M. J. F. Digonnet, and G. S. Kino, "Measurement of the dc Kerr and electrostrictive phase modulation in silica," J. Opt. Soc. Am. B 18, 187, (2001)

20. D. Faccio, V. Pruneri, and P. G. Kazanksy, "Dynamics of the second order nonlinearity in thermally poled silica glass," Appl. Phys. Lett. 79, 2687 (2001)

21. N. Boling, A. Glass, and A. Owyoung, "Empirical relationships for predicting nonlinear refractive index changes in optical solids," IEEE J. Quant. Electron. 14, 601 (1978)

22. A. Ozcan, M. J. F. Digonnet, and G. S. Kino, "Simplified inverse Fourier transform technique to measure optical nonlinearity profiles using reference sample," Electron. Lett. 40, 551 (2004)

23. Y. Quiquempois, G. Martinelli, P. Dutherage, P. Bernage, P. and M. Douay, "Localisation of the induced second-order non-linearity within Infrasil and Suprasil thermally poled glasses," Opt. Comm. 176, 479 (2000)

24. A. Kameyama, A. Yokotani, K. Kurosawa, "Generation and erasure of second-order optical nonlinearities in thermally poled silica glasses by control of point defects," J. Opt. Soc. Am. B 19, 2376 (2002)

25. P. Thamboon and D. M. Krol, "Second-order optical nonlinearities in thermally poled phosphate glasses," J. Appl. Phys. 93, 32 (2003)

26. R. T. Crosswell, A. Reisman, D. L. Simpson, D. Temple, and C. K. Williams, "Planarization processes and applications: III. As-deposited and annealed film properties," J. Electrochem. Soc. 147, 1513 (2000)

CHAPTER 5: CHARACTERIZATION OF ULTRASHORT OPTICAL PULSES: SPECTRAL INTERFEROMETRY USING MINIMUM-PHASE BASED ALGORITHM (SIMBA)

This chapter describes the characterization of ultrashort optical pulses (sub picosecond duration) using a powerful tool, which we have called Spectral Interferometry using Minimum-phase Based Algorithms (SIMBA). The classical spectral interferometry involves forming a pulse sequence consisting of a reference pulse followed by the sample pulse to be characterized, and measuring the power spectrum of this sequence with an optical spectrum analyzer (OSA). To fully characterize an unknown sample pulse, the classical approach requires a known reference pulse. We demonstrate that if the reference pulse electric field amplitude is made larger than the unknown pulse amplitude by a factor of >5-10 and also if the reference pulse temporal width is narrower than the temporal width of the unknown sample pulse by a factor of >~5, then using a minimum phase based processing, the complex electric field of the sample pulse can be accurately recovered *without* the need for a known reference pulse, which reduces the measurement time and complexity significantly. To our knowledge, this is the first time the concept of minimum-phase functions has been applied to this problem. Experimental spectral interferometry curves reported in this chapter were provided by David N. Fittinghoff of Lawrence Livermore National Laboratory, (Fig. 27), and by Selcuk Akturk of Georgia Institute of Technology, (Fig. 29). All the relevant data analysis together with the principles of theory were developed by Aydogan Ozcan under the supervision of Gordon S. Kino and Michel J. F. Digonnet.

5.1 INTRODUCTION

Ultra-short optical pulses with a sub-picosecond time scale play a key role in many important applications such as medical imaging, surgery, micro-machining, optical communication, and 3D optical waveguide fabrication.[1-5] In almost all of these applications, knowledge of the complex electric-field temporal profile, $e(t)$, of the laser pulse is critical (the physical electric-field oscillations of the optical field are related to

$e(t)$ by: $E(t) = \text{Re}\,al\{e(t) \cdot \exp(j \cdot \omega_c \cdot t)\}$, where ω_c is the center angular frequency of the laser spectrum). For this purpose, over the last decade many techniques have been developed to characterize ultra-short pulses.[6-18] Most of these techniques involve employing nonlinear optics, i.e., typically use a thin nonlinear crystal. One of the earliest of these nonlinear characterization efforts was the classical intensity auto-correlator.[6] The fundamental limitation with this early technology is that (1) it cannot yield a unique solution to the intensity profile of an ultrashort pulse; and (2) it does not provide any information related to the phase spectrum of the ultrashort pulse. Since the discovery of this rather old and limited technique, much more sophisticated and powerful techniques were invented. Some of the well-known powerful nonlinear techniques are frequency-resolved optical gating (FROG),[8] spectral phase interferometry for direct electric-field reconstruction (SPIDER),[12] spectrally resolved cross-correlation (XFROG),[15] and phase and intensity from cross-correlation and spectrum only (PICASO).[17] Because the nonlinear process is generally weak, these techniques tend to require high peak powers and are generally not suitable for characterizing weak pulses. Linear techniques[9-11,13-14] were conceived in part to eliminate this power limitation. A well known example of linear techniques is spectral interferometry (SI), which uses a linear detection system, such as an optical spectrum analyzer (OSA), to record in the frequency domain the interference between the sample pulse to be characterized and a reference pulse.[9-11] Temporal analysis by dispersing a pair of light e-fields (TADPOLE)[10] is one of the most popular SI techniques: the reference pulse is first fully characterized using a FROG set-up, then an OSA is used to measure the power spectra of the sample pulse and of a pulse sequence formed by delaying the reference pulse with respect to the sample pulse. These *three* measurements enable the recovery of the full complex electric field of the sample pulse, even if this pulse is very weak.[10] Note that all SI-based techniques require a fully characterized reference pulse.[9-11, 13]

In this chapter, we demonstrate a different approach to spectral interferometry, which we refer to as Spectral Interferometry using Minimum-phase Based Algorithms (SIMBA). SIMBA relies on the same set-up as the classical SI requires and therefore shares all the benefits of SI such as being a linear technique that can characterize ultraweak pulses, having a simple measurement set-up that does not contain any moving parts, being able to differentiate an ultrashort pulse from its time-reversed replica, etc. We demonstrate that under certain set of conditions, there is a simpler and more powerful way of processing the SI data, i.e., the recorded optical power spectrum, to recover the unknown sample pulse's complex electric field. The classical SI has one fundamental requirement to characterize an unknown sample pulse using a *known* reference pulse: the bandwidth of the reference pulse has to cover roughly the bandwidth of the sample pulse to be characterized. SIMBA has two more additional requirements on the top of this classical SI requirement: (1) the maximum amplitude of the reference pulse electric field has to be larger than the maximum amplitude of the sample pulse to be characterized by e.g., $>\sim$5-10 times; and (2) the temporal width of the reference pulse has to be narrower than the temporal width of the sample pulse by typically $>\sim$5 times. Under these additional constraints, we demonstrate that SIMBA can recover the complex electric field profile of the sample pulse using a *single* OSA measurement, *without additional knowledge of the reference pulse profile*. We should immediately note that the first requirement of SIMBA is actually not a limiting factor, since it naturally occurs in characterization of weak ultrashort pulses using a stronger reference pulse. Furthermore, if need be, the sample pulse can simply be attenuated to achieve the desired power ratio between the reference and sample pulses. The second requirement of SIMBA, as will be discussed later on, makes our technique especially suitable to characterize highly chirped weak ultrashort pulses, i.e., weak pulses that are far away from being transform-limited, where a transform-limited pulse is defined as the pulse that has the shortest temporal width corresponding to a given magnitude spectrum. Also noteworthy is that, in applications like pump-probe experiments, after going through the experiment under investigation, the pulses usually acquire complicated temporal structures, directly increasing the pulse duration. Therefore, a portion of the input pulse can easily satisfy the temporal width condition for the reference pulse, and can therefore be used to measure the output pulse of the pump-probe experiment. Since SIMBA does not require the electric field profile of the reference pulse, from now on the reference pulse of SIMBA will be referred to as the 'dummy' pulse.

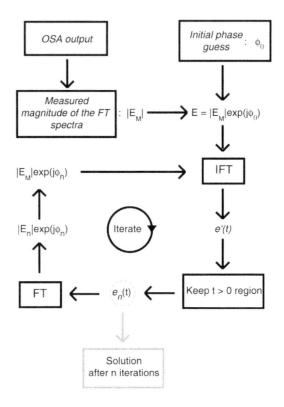

Fig. 1. General block diagram of the iterative error reduction algorithm applied to recover an MPF from its measured FT magnitude spectrum.

The crux of SIMBA is that by construction (a large dummy pulse followed by a weaker sample pulse), the pulse sequence is close to a minimum-phase function (MPF), which means that it is possible to recover its temporal profile from the magnitude of its Fourier transform (i.e., its measured power spectrum) *alone,* either analytically or iteratively.[19-21]. As described below, this recovery is carried out numerically with a simple iterative algorithm that takes only seconds on a 500-MHz computer using MATLAB 5. The reasons for choosing the iterative approach over the analytical approach are (1) simplicity of its numerical evaluation, and (2) better noise performance. With a faster computer and programming tool, this technique, like several other techniques including FROG, TADPOLE or SPIDER, has the capacity to provide real-time dynamic measurements of a laser pulse profile that satisfies the above-mentioned conditions. To our knowledge, this is the first time that the concept of minimum phase functions has been applied to the characterization of optical pulses.

5.2 MINIMUM PHASE FUNCTIONS AND THEIR IMPLICATIONS FOR ULTRA-SHORT OPTICAL PULSE CHARACTERIZATION

It is well known that, in general, a one-dimensional function cannot be recovered from the knowledge of its FT magnitude alone. However, there are exceptions to this rule, namely families of functions for which the FT phase can be recovered from the FT magnitude alone, and visa versa. As already shown in Chapter 2, one important such family is minimum-phase functions (MPFs).[19] The FT phase of an MPF can always be reconstructed from its FT amplitude. This reconstruction can, in principle, be done by taking the Hilbert transform of the logarithm of the function's FT magnitude. For reasons explained in Chapter 2, such as difficulties in its numerical evaluation, particularly in phase unwrapping,[20] and higher noise sensitivity, this direct approach is not the preferred solution. Instead, we use an iterative error-reduction algorithm, for example the Fienup[22] or the Gerchberg-Saxton[23] algorithm. A general block diagram of these iterative algorithms, specifically tailored for the application of ultrashort pulse complex electric field characterization, is shown in Fig. 1. Given a complex MPF, $e(t)$, the only quantity that is fed into the algorithm is the FT magnitude spectrum of $e(t)$, i.e., $|E_M(f)|$, where the subscript M denotes that this spectrum is a measured quantity. There is an important difference between the previous version of the iterative error-reduction algorithm presented in Chapter 3, and the current version shown in Fig. 1: in Chapter 3, the function of interest, i.e., the nonlinearity depth profile of thin films, was known to be a real quantity. However, the function of interest for this chapter, $e(t)$, is a complex function. Therefore, unlike in Chapter 3, at each iteration, only the causality principle can be forced on the solution, by setting to zero all values of $e'(t)$ for $t < 0$. Because the constraint in this case is weaker than the constraint applied in Chapter 3, the recovery is much more challenging. It should also be emphasized that if $e(t)$ were known to be limited in time, for example to be less than 100 fs long, we could also insert zeros for $t >$ 100 fs, to speed up convergence.

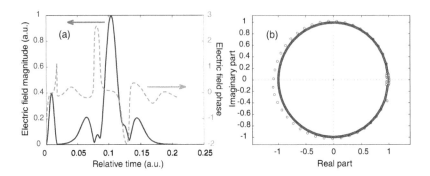

Fig. 2 (a) A sequence of complex electric field magnitude and phase, (b) pole-zero plot of the z-transform of the sequence shown in (a). Zeros are shown with the circles. Since there are many zeros outside the unit circle, the function shown in (a) is not an MPF.

In Chapter 2, it was illustrated with numerical examples that MPF condition was strictly related to the amplitude of the function at the origin. Following the intuition developed in Chapter 2, any profile with a *dominant* peak around $t = 0$ (i.e., close to the origin) will be either a minimum-phase function or close to one, and thus will work *extremely well* with the iterative error-reduction algorithm outlined in Fig. 1. To further illustrate the importance of a dominant peak close to the origin, we examined the exemplary complex electric-field function shown in Fig. 2(a). The magnitude of this causal function has four peaks. The first one (close to the origin $t = 0$) has a magnitude of 0.4, and the dominant peak (around $t = 0.1$) has a magnitude of 1.0. Since the dominant peak is not the one closest to the origin, this function is not an MPF. This can be verified by the pole-zero plot of the sequence's z-transform, shown in Fig. 2(b): many zeros of the z-transform lie outside the unit circle. Because the sequence shown in Fig. 2(a) is not an MPF, the phase and magnitude of its FT cannot be accurately related by the Hilbert transform or by iterative error-correction algorithms. This is illustrated in Fig. 3, which shows the complex electric field function obtained by applying the iterative algorithm of Fig. 1 to the FT magnitude of Fig. 2(a). Both the recovered phase and amplitude functions (dashed curves) are substantially different from the original functions (solid curves, which are the same as in Fig. 2(a)). It is significant that the function recovered by the error-reduction algorithm of Fig. 1 exhibits a large peak in its amplitude near $t = 0$ as shown in Fig. 3(a) with the dot-dashed curve: the reason is that the algorithm converges to *the* minimum phase function associated with the original FT magnitude spectrum, which must have a dominant peak near the origin.

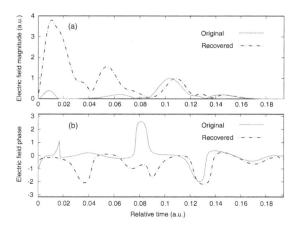

Fig. 3. (a) Magnitude and (b) phase recovered by applying the iterative error-reduction algorithm of Fig. 1 to the FT *magnitude* of the complex electric-field function shown in Fig. 2(a).

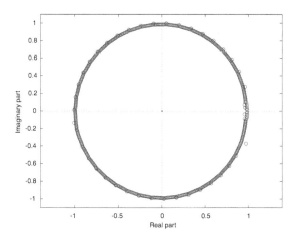

Fig. 4. Pole-zero plot of the z-transform of the sequence shown in Fig. 2(a), when the amplitude of the first peak is increased to 50. Zeros are shown as circles. Since almost all of the zeros of the z-transform are either inside or very close to the unit circle, this sequence is very close to an MPF.

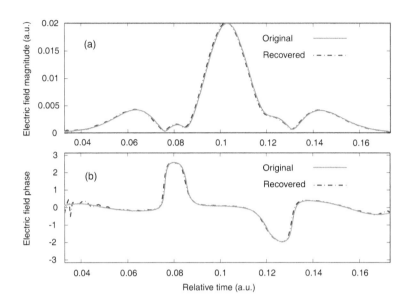

Fig. 5. (a) Magnitude and (b) phase recovered by applying the Fienup algorithm to the FT *magnitude* of the complex electric field function of Fig. 2(a) when the amplitude of the first peak is increased to 50.

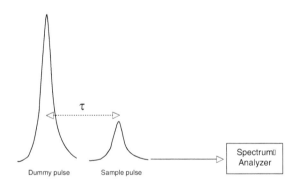

Dummy pulse   Sample pulse

Spectrum
Analyzer

Fig. 6. SIMBA requires the same set-up as the classical SI requires.

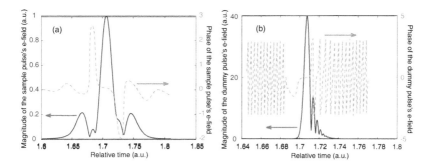

Fig. 7. Temporal profile of the complex electric field of (a) the sample pulse and (b) the dummy pulse.

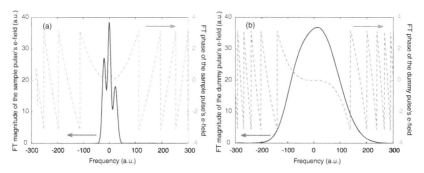

Fig. 8. Calculated FT magnitude and phase spectra of (a) the sample and (b) dummy pulses of Fig. 7.

To understand the foundations of SIMBA, we now examine what happens when the magnitude of the first peak in Fig. 2(a) is increased from 0.4 to a large value, for example 50 (without changing the phase in Fig. 2(a)), so that it becomes the dominant peak. The pole-zero plot of the new sequence (Fig. 4) shows that almost all of the zeros of its z-transform are now either in or very close to the unit circle. Increasing the first peak magnitude pushes all the zeros of the function's z-transform towards the unit circle, i.e., it makes the new sequence closer to a true MPF. Since this new sequence is very close to an MPF, the phase and magnitude of its FT are accurately related by the Hilbert transform or by iterative error-reduction algorithms. To illustrate this point, we plotted in Fig. 5 the complex function recovered by applying the iterative algorithm of Fig. 1 to the FT magnitude of the new sequence. As expected, the recovery is excellent.

5.3 CHARACTERIZATION OF ULTRA-SHORT PULSES USING MINIMUM PHASE FUNCTIONS

Based on the foregoing treatment, SIMBA determines the complex electric field temporal profile of an ultrashort pulse by placing a strong reference pulse time ahead of this pulse (Fig. 6), then sending this sequence into an OSA to measure the square of the FT magnitude of the complex sequence. As explained above, because the addition of a strong dummy pulse makes the complex pulse sequence close to an MPF, it is now possible to recover the complex sample pulse profile from the measured spectrum, using an error-reduction algorithm such as the one shown in Fig. 1.

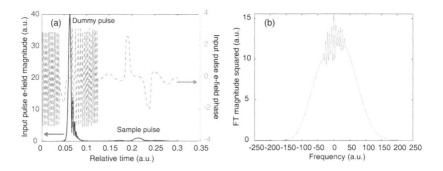

Fig. 9. (a) Complex electric field of the pulse sequence formed by delaying the sample pulse in time with respect to the stronger dummy pulse. The ratio of the two pulses' electric field magnitudes was chosen to be 40. (b) Power spectrum (i.e., square of the FT magnitude) of the complex electric field shown in (a).

To demonstrate the SIMBA technique step by step, we applied it to the exemplary sample pulse shown in Fig. 7(a). The solid curve is the amplitude of the pulse's temporal electric field profile, and the dashed curve is its phase. This pulse was selected arbitrarily, except that: (1) we included a strong second-order phase in its FT (Fig. 8(a)), a case that makes it more difficult to retrieve the pulse profile; and (2) the phase and amplitude were selected so that the pulse's FT magnitude spectrum, calculated numerically and shown in Fig. 8(a), resembles the spectrum of typical practical pulses. Figure 9(b) shows the amplitude and phase of the dummy pulse. The calculated FT spectrum of this dummy pulse is plotted in Fig. 8(b). The dummy pulse shape was also selected arbitrarily, with a large amount of third-order phase in its FT (Fig. 8(b)); this is responsible for the oscillations in the tail of the pulse amplitude (Fig. 7(b)). For reasons explained above, the peak amplitude of the dummy pulse electric field was taken to be much larger than the sample pulse peak amplitude (by a factor of 40, or 1600 in peak power).

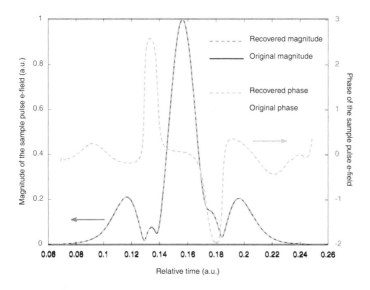

Fig. 10. The recovered complex electric field temporal profile of the weak sample pulse shown in Fig. 9. The recovered quantities are shown as dashed curves; the actual complex field (the same as in Fig. 9(a)) is shown as solid curves.

Next, the sample pulse was delayed in time by τ with respect to the dummy pulse to form the pulse sequence shown in Fig. 9(a), which is by construction close to an MPF. The minimum constraint on τ is that it must be large enough that the two pulses do not overlap. This constraint is not as strict as for other SI techniques. All other SI techniques require a larger minimum delay than SIMBA in order to avoid aliasing in the inverse FT domain, which would make the recovery impossible. (For a relevant discussion on SI requirements refer to Chapter 3.) In the case of SIMBA, aliasing can be present because it does not affect the recovery process. On the other hand, the delay τ should also not be too large for the same reason as in other SI techniques: a large delay results in high-frequency oscillations in the measured spectrum of the pulse sequence, which then requires a higher resolution OSA. Sending this pulse sequence into an OSA yields the square of the FT magnitude of the complex electric field temporal profile. This calculated spectrum is shown in Fig. 9(b). The oscillations present around the center of the spectrum are due to the interference between the two pulses' electric fields.

Figure 9(b) contains all the necessary information to recover the sample pulse's complex electric field. This is done by applying the Fienup algorithm shown in Fig. 1 to $|E_M(f)|$, i.e., the *square root* of the spectrum of Fig. 9(b). The amplitude and phase of the electric field of the sample pulse obtained by this process are plotted as dashed curves in Fig. 10. A comparison with the amplitude and phase of the original pulse, reproduced from Fig. 7(a) as solid curves, shows that both the amplitude and phase components of the recovered pulse are virtually indistinguishable from the original pulse components. The beauty of this technique is that it recovers the complex electric field of an optical pulse from a *single FT magnitude measurement*, and that it does so without the need for any additional information about the dummy pulse. This outstanding result required a computation time of only a few seconds, using MATLAB 5 on a 500-MHz computer. The number of data points used to simulate the measured FT magnitude (Fig. 9(b)) was limited to ~1500. To increase the resolution and speed of the processing (which involves fast FT routines), the total number of points was increased to 2^{14} by zero padding. Real-time characterization of ultra-short pulses using SIMBA is therefore possible by using a much faster programming environment such as C++. As noted above, this recovery could be done using the analytical Hilbert transform[19] instead of an iterative approach, although this method could be more susceptible to noise.

Since SIMBA does not record the arrival times of the input pulses, the recovered profile exhibits a time shift compared to the actual pulse. (This shift is not visible in Fig. 10 because for comparison purposes, the recovered pulse was shifted to match the original pulse.) This feature is, of course, common to all existing recovery techniques, and is inconsequential. In the recovered phase, the slight deviation (also inconsequential), especially toward the edges of Fig. 10, is primarily due to the very weak intensity of the pulse at those times, which makes the phase recovery less accurate. In the limiting case, at the times when the pulse intensity goes to zero, the recovery of the exact phase becomes almost impossible, but since the phase of a zero field is meaningless, this limitation is inconsequential. This same phenomenon is also present in other techniques, e.g., FROG, TADPOLE, and SPIDER.

We also checked what would happen if time-reversal were applied to either one or both of the pulses. In all three cases, the recovery was as good as the recovery shown in Fig. 10, i.e., SIMBA conveniently differentiates between a pulse and its time-reversed version. This attribute is an important improvement over some of the widely used techniques (such as second harmonic FROG), which cannot differentiate a pulse from its time-reversed replica, and hence require additional information regarding the pulse to remove this ambiguity.[1]

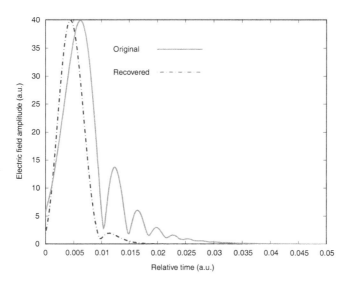

Fig. 11. Magnitude of the complex electric field temporal profile of the original dummy pulse (solid curve) and of the recovered dummy pulse (dashed curve). The unsatisfactory recovery of the dummy pulse is inconsequential, since it is not the target pulse that needs to be characterized. The sample pulse starts at $t > 0.05$ and is not shown.

It is interesting to note that the dummy pulse is generally not recovered well (which is, of course, inconsequential). This is illustrated by the recovered magnitude of the dummy pulse used in the recovery of Fig. 10, which is reproduced in Fig. 11, as well as by the original dummy pulse (solid curve, reproduced from Fig. 9(a)). Most of the significant features of the original dummy profile, such as the oscillations in the tail, are washed out in the recovered dummy pulse profile. This behavior is expected because the pulse sequence is *close* to an MPF but not a true MPF. Consequently, the recovery algorithm, which always converges to a true MPF, produces a sequence that is perforce somewhat different from the original sequence. Figure 11 shows that almost all of the differences between the recovered and original profiles occur around the first dominant peak (i.e., the dummy pulse). This important feature can be explained by the fact that the minimum phase condition is strictly related to the dominant peak's shape and magnitude. Specifically, for a function to be a true MPF, the rise time of its dominant peak at the origin ($t = 0$ in this case) must be very sharp. Since this condition cannot be met perfectly with practical dummy pulses in the laboratory, the constructed pulse sequence is not a true MPF. On the other hand, the shape of the sample pulse has little bearing on whether the sequence is a true MPF. In a simplistic view, the recovery of the dummy pulse is sacrificed (which is inconsequential) to achieve a very good recovery for the following weaker sample pulse.

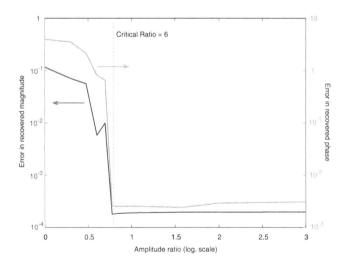

Fig. 12. Error in the recovered electric field magnitude and phase as a function of the ratio of the peak magnitude of the dummy pulse to the peak magnitude of the sample pulse. The error drops to an insignificant level above a critical ratio of ~6.

The parameter that influences the accuracy of the recovery most strongly is the magnitude of the dummy pulse compared to the sample pulse magnitude. For the recovery results shown in Fig. 10, the ratio of amplitudes was chosen to be 40. To investigate the impact of this ratio on the recovery accuracy, we carried out the same simulation as Figs. 7-10 for different dummy to sample pulse amplitude ratios, and plotted the error in the recovered sample pulse profile as a function of this ratio (see Fig. 12). The error was defined as $\dfrac{\int \left| f(t) - \hat{f}(t) \right|^2 dt}{\int \left| f(t) \right|^2 dt}$, where $f(t)$ and $\hat{f}(t)$ are the original and the recovered quantities, respectively, and where the integrals were calculated over the time duration of the sample pulse only. Figure 12 demonstrates that at a critical ratio of ~6, the error in both the phase and the magnitude drops dramatically. Above this ratio the error is roughly constant and less than ~2 10^{-4}. Through trial and error we have found that this critical ratio depends on the functional form of both pulses, and it typically ranges between ~5 and ~15. To be on the safe side, choosing a ratio greater than 20–30 will work well in most cases. Furthermore, if need be, the convergence of the technique can be checked by carrying out the spectral measurement for two ratio values, e.g., 25 and 50, and making sure that the difference between the two solutions is negligible. Another important result of Fig. 12 is that the recovery remains equally good with ratios as large as 1000. This is especially important for the detection of ultra weak pulses, i.e., SIMBA can characterize an ultrashort pulse that is at least 1 million times weaker in peak power than the leading dummy pulse.

Next we look at the issue of noise sensitivity, i.e., how measurement errors and noise in the power spectrum affect the accuracy of the profiles recovered with SIMBA. For this purpose, we took an arbitrary dummy-sample pulse sequence (with a peak amplitude ratio of 13), calculated the square of its theoretical FT magnitude (dashed curve in Fig. 13), and multiplied this spectrum by a uniform random noise with a 20% peak-to-peak amplitude and an average of unity (solid curve in Fig. 13). We then applied SIMBA to each spectrum and compared the sample pulse profile recovered from the noise-free spectrum and from the noisy spectrum. The two recovered profiles are shown in Fig. 14. The recovery is still quite good: in spite of the large measurement noise, the mean error in the recovered pulse intensity is less than 1.5%. Simulations also show that the mean error in the recovered profile is proportional to the error in the spectrum, as expected. This shows that SIMBA works well even with fairly noisy measurements. The noise sensitivity is affected by the ratio of the dummy to sample pulse magnitudes. If the main source of noise in the OSA measurement system is proportional to the input power, as assumed above, then the larger the dummy pulse, the stronger the noise in the measured spectrum, and the stronger the error in the recovered sample pulse profile. To maximize the accuracy of the recovered profiles in the presence of noisy measurements, it is therefore preferable to select an amplitude ratio close to the critical ratio, e.g., in the range of ~5 to ~15 (see Fig. 12). This is the reason for using an amplitude ratio of 13 in Fig. 13. This choice ensures both accurate convergence of the iterative algorithm and reduced sensitivity to measurement noise. In practice the optimum amplitude ratio can be found by comparing the recovery results of a few different power ratio values. The smallest ratio after which the average difference between the recovery results do not change defines the critical power ratio that ensures the convergence.

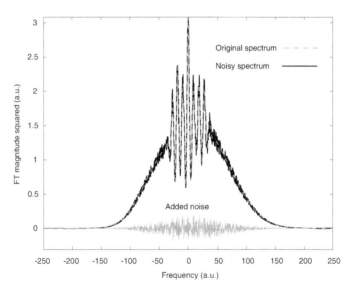

Fig. 13. Noise-free and noisy FT magnitude square of a pulse sequence (see text for details) used to illustrate the impact of noise on the recovered sample profile.

The accuracy of SIMBA is also affected by the frequency bandwidths of the two pulses. Here, we define the bandwidth as the full width of the FT magnitude spectrum at

10% of its maximum value. The effect of bandwidth is related to the last requirement of SIMBA: the temporal width of the dummy pulse has to be narrower than the temporal width of the sample pulse, by >~2-5 times. For two pulses (dummy and sample) that have roughly the same time-bandwidth product, the effect of relative bandwidths of the pulses becomes more important for SIMBA. As in all other SI techniques, the bandwidth of the dummy pulse in SIMBA needs to cover at least the bandwidth of the sample pulse. In the numerical example of Fig. 8, the bandwidth of the dummy pulse was ~4.5 times that of the sample pulse. This can be seen in Fig. 8, but also in Fig. 9(b), where the narrower band in which the interference fringes occur represents roughly the frequency range of the sample pulse.

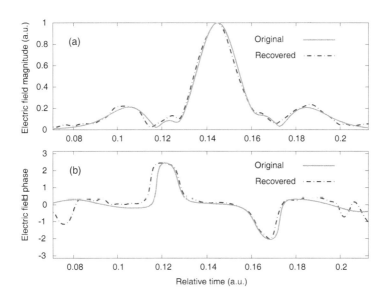

Fig. 14. (a) Magnitude and (b) phase of the electric field of the sample pulse recovered from the noisy FT spectrum shown in Fig. 13.

To evaluate the effect of bandwidth ratio on the accuracy of the method, we carried out a new numerical simulation with a bandwidth ratio of ~2. The sample and dummy electric-field pulses used in this simulation are plotted in Fig. 15, and their FT spectra in Fig. 16. In this numerical example, the temporal width of the dummy pulse is chosen to be ~2.4 times narrower than the temporal width of the sample pulse. A temporal width ratio of 2.4 together with a bandwidth ratio of 2 implies that the time-bandwidth product of the dummy pulse roughly matches that of the sample pulse. We have included strong third-order and second-order phase in the FT spectra of the sample and dummy pulses, respectively (the reverse of the example used in Fig. 8). As a result, the temporal profiles of the two pulses are quite different from the previous example (compare Figs. 9 and 15). The electric field of the pulse sequence formed by delaying the two pulses of Fig. 15 is plotted in Fig. 17(a). In this case, the amplitude ratio of the two pulses was chosen to be 30. The computed square of the FT magnitude of this sequence is shown in Fig. 17(b).

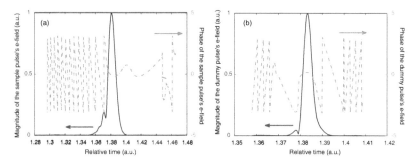

Fig. 15. Temporal profile of the normalized complex electric field corresponding to (a) the sample and (b) the dummy pulses. The dummy pulse is temporally narrower than the sample pulse by a factor of ~2.4.

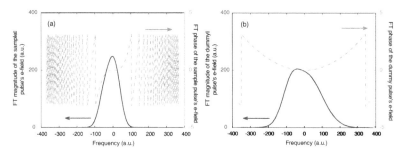

Fig. 16. FT magnitude and phase spectra of the (a) sample and (b) dummy pulses. The ratio of the bandwidth of the dummy pulse to the bandwidth of the sample pulse is ~2.

The sample pulse recovered by applying SIMBA to Fig. 17(b) (dashed curves in Fig. 18) is again in very good agreement with the original pulse (solid curves in Fig. 18).

This result demonstrates that in the case, where the time-bandwidth products of the dummy and sample pulses are comparable, a bandwidth ratio of ~2 is still high enough for a reliable recovery. To further investigate the effect of relative bandwidth of the sample and dummy pulses on the recovery, we ran a number of simulations where the bandwidth ratio of the dummy pulse to the sample pulse was varied from ~0.87 to ~2.7, the results of which are shown in Fig. 19. In this simulation, a fixed value of 30 was chosen for the ratio of the maximum amplitude of the dummy pulse to the sample pulse. Furthermore, in each run, the time-bandwidth products of the dummy and sample pulses were preserved, in other words their spectra were simply changed without affecting their functional forms. The results of this simulation (Fig. 19) revealed that reducing the bandwidth ratio to less than 1 would introduce a noticeable error in the recovered profile. This result is expected: if the bandwidth of the dummy pulse is narrower than the bandwidth of the sample pulse, some of the high frequency components in the FT magnitude spectrum (e.g., see Fig. 17(b)) will be missing, and since these oscillations carry information regarding the sample pulse, it will no longer be possible to accurately recover the latter. A minimum bandwidth ratio of at least 1 is required for a good recovery. This minimum bandwidth requirement is not specific to our technique; all other SI techniques require a reference pulse with a broader spectrum than the ultrashort pulses to be characterized. Note that with SIMBA, there is no maximum bandwidth ratio requirement: the dummy pulse bandwidth can be as much as 1000 times wider than the sample pulse bandwidth. In practice, the maximum dummy pulse bandwidth will be imposed by the available laser. Note in Fig. 18 the slight dc offset between the recovered and the original phase spectra. None of the existing techniques, including SIMBA, can recover this dc phase component, which corresponds physically to the relative phase of the electric-field oscillations under the complex electric-field envelope $e(t)$. For many applications, this offset is inconsequential.

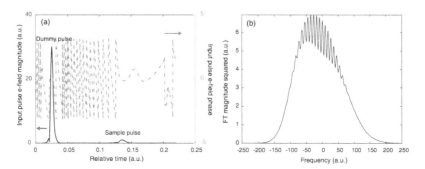

Fig. 17. (a) Complex electric field of the pulse sequence formed by delaying a sample pulse with respect to a dummy pulse. The amplitude ratio of the electric field of the two pulses was chosen to be 30. (b) Square of the FT *magnitude* of the complex electric field shown in (a).

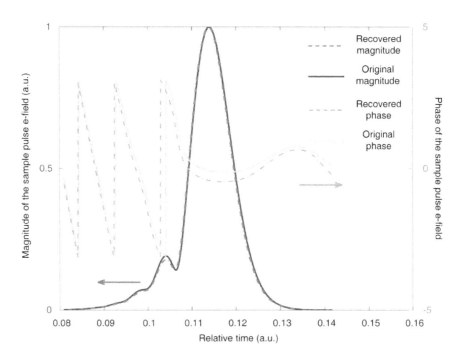

Fig. 18. Recovered complex electric field temporal profile of the sample pulse of Fig. 17(a).

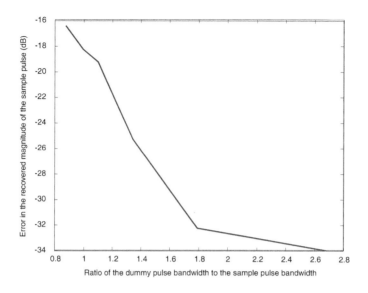

Fig. 19. Error, defined in *10 log* of the recovered magnitude of the sample pulse as a function of the ratio between the dummy pulse bandwidth and the sample pulse bandwidth.

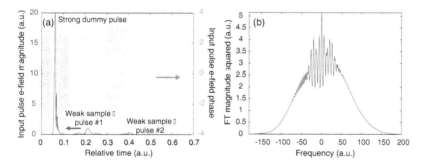

Fig. 20. (a) Complex electric field of the pulse sequence formed by delaying two different sample pulses with respect to a dummy pulse. The relative maximum electric field amplitudes of these three pulses are 20, 1, and 1/3, respectively. (b) Square of the FT magnitude of the complex electric field shown in (a).

For cases where the bandwidths of the sample and dummy pulses are comparable, which naturally occurs in many experiments involving *linear* optics, if the spectral phase of the dummy pulse (ϕ_f) is of the same order of magnitude as the spectral phase of the sample pulse (ϕ_g), then the temporal width requirement of SIMBA is violated. This

113

directly implies that, as mentioned earlier, SIMBA is particularly suitable for characterizing highly dispersed ultrashort pulses, which are quite far away from being transform-limited. In many cases, these highly chirped pulses actually result from the interaction of a short pulse with an experimental set-up, such as in the pump-probe experiments. Therefore, in most pump-probe experiments, the short pump pulse can itself serve as the dummy pulse of SIMBA. In other cases, where this is not possible, for a given sample pulse, a dummy pulse that satisfies the temporal width requirement of SIMBA can be generated from the sample pulse itself in two different ways. The first method relies on nonlinear pulse compressors,[26-27] whereas the second method relies on linear pulse compressors[1]. Nonlinear pulse compressors can increase the bandwidth of the input sample pulse such that the compressed output pulse can act as the dummy pulse required by SIMBA. However this approach makes SIMBA a nonlinear technique, which takes away an important motivation of SIMBA: being a linear technique that can characterize ultraweak pulses. For this reason, the second approach, which relies on linear pulse compressors, such as a pair of gratings or prisms is preferred. In this second class of linear pulse compressors, the time-bandwidth product of the input pulse is reduced (with a compression ratio of ~5-10) without changing the bandwidth of input pulse. The new compressed pulse can itself serve as the dummy pulse to characterize the sample pulse. The function of the pulse compressor is simply to satisfy the third condition of SIMBA, i.e., to make the pulse width of the dummy pulse narrower (e.g., by a factor of $>$~5) than the pulse width of the sample pulse. Another way of looking at the same phenomenon is that the large spectral phase, ϕ_g, of the highly dispersed sample pulse is reduced by the linear pulse compressor, such that the time-bandwidth product of the compressed sample pulse, which now acts as a dummy pulse, becomes smaller than the time-bandwidth product of the initial sample pulse. Therefore, after the linear pulse compressor $\phi_f \ll \phi_g$ is satisfied. However, we should also note that SIMBA does *not* require a transform-limited dummy pulse. Actually *none* of the pulses shown in this chapter are transform-limited.

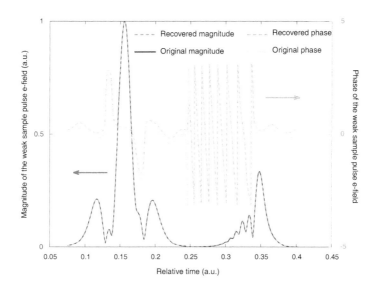

Fig. 21. Simultaneous recovery of two sample pulses' electric fields using a single FT magnitude spectrum.

One of the other benefits of SIMBA is that it can also characterize the complex electric field profile of a series of laser pulses (as might be generated, for example, by multiple laser sources) with a single spectrum measurement. To illustrate this point, consider as an example a series of two sample pulses formed by delaying two different ultrashort laser pulses, as shown in Fig. 20(a) (for a magnified view see Fig. 21). The leading dummy pulse in Fig. 20(a) is chosen to be the same as in Fig. 7(b). The relative maximum electric field amplitudes of these three pulses were chosen to be 20, 1 and 1/3, respectively. (The recovery results were independent of these relative amplitudes; for example, relative amplitudes of 40, 1, 1 or 30, 1, 1/2 gave similar results.) The computed square of the FT magnitude of the complex profile of Fig. 20(a) is plotted in Fig. 20(b). Applying the same iterative error-reduction algorithm as before to Fig. 20(b) allowed us to simultaneously recover the complex electric field profile of both sample pulses (dashed curves in Fig. 21). The recovery is as good as in the previous examples. This is a very powerful result: using a single spectrum measurement, we have simultaneously recovered the full complex electric fields of two different ultrashort pulses. Equally good recoveries are obtained when the two pulses have different profiles.

Note that again, there is a small inconsequential dc offset in the recovered phase spectrum, and that, in the time interval between the two sample pulses, the error in the recovered phase spectrum is simply due to the fact that the magnitude of the electric field in that interval is very close or equal to zero, as discussed above.

SIMBA can characterize series containing many more than two individual pulses. However, when the number of pulses is too large, the oscillations in the FT magnitude arising from multiple interferences between the pulses become so rapid that a higher resolution OSA is required. Therefore, the number of pulses that can be simultaneously characterized depends on the resolution of the OSA, together with the temporal profiles of the dummy and sample pulses.

We would like to mention that various ultrashort pulse shaping techniques[28-29] can be used to modify the temporal profile of the dummy pulse in order to achieve an absolutely *true* MPF for the pulse sequence's electric field. This could potentially improve the recovery speed of SIMBA dramatically. In principle, by using a true MPF, the algorithm can converge in less than e.g., 5 iterations, cutting down the computation time to a fraction of a second, even in a relatively slow programming environment such as MATLAB 5.

5.4 SIMBA VS. SI

The goal of this section is to emphasize the differences between SIMBA and the classical SI. For this purpose, let us focus on an arbitrary pulse sequence $s(t) = f(t) + g(t - \tau)$, where $f(t)$ and $g(t)$ represent the reference (dummy) and sample pulses' complex electric field envelopes, respectively.

The detected signal in all SI based techniques, including SIMBA, will always be proportional to the square of the Fourier transform (FT) magnitude of the input pulse sequence, $s(t)$, i.e.:

$$|S(f)|^2 = |F(f)|^2 + |G(f)|^2 + 2|F(f)||G(f)|cos(\phi_g - \phi_f - 2\pi f\tau) \qquad (1)$$

where $S(f)$, $F(f) = |F(f)| \cdot exp(j \cdot \phi_f(f))$ and $G(f) = |G(f)| \cdot exp(j \cdot \phi_g(f))$ define the FT's of $s(t)$, $f(t)$ and $g(t)$, respectively. In the classical SI, the direct inverse FT (IFT) of $|S(f)|^2$ is taken, which after appropriate filtering of the term around $t = \tau$, yields the complex correlation of $f(t)$ with $g(t)$, i.e.,

$$C_{SI}(t) = g(t) * f(t) = IFT \left\{ F(f) |G(f)| exp(j(\phi_g - \phi_f)) \right\} \quad (2)$$

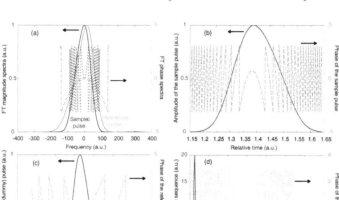

Fig. 22. (a)FT magnitude and phase spectrum of the reference and sample pulses; (b) temporal profile of the sample pulse; (c) temporal profile of the reference pulse; and (d) the pulse sequence formed with the reference and sample pulses.

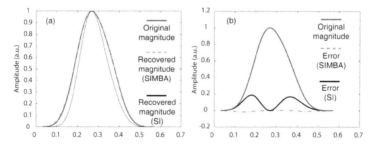

Fig. 23. (a) Recovery results for the amplitude of the sample pulse; and (b) error in recovery.

117

Eq. (2) is all the information that the classical IFT based SI approach can yield without a known reference pulse. The fundamental limitation of this classical SI approach is that, if the reference pulse information is *not* known, in general $C_{SI}(t) = g(t) * f(t)$ is quite different from $g(t)$. To give an idea, for the two pulses, $g(t)$ and $f(t)$, shown in Figs. 22(b) and 22(c), respectively, the output of the classical SI is shown in Fig. 23(a). For this simulation a ratio 20 was used between the reference and sample pulse peak amplitudes (Fig. 22(d)). A comparison of $C_{SI}(t) = g(t) * f(t)$ with $g(t)$ shows the error to be quite high (Fig. 23(b)). To further illustrate the limitation of the classical SI approach, let us give a second example, where $g(t)$ and $f(t)$ are chosen as shown in Figs. 24(b) and 24(c), respectively. Using a ratio of ~40 in the formed pulse sequence, the recovery using the classical IFT based SI approach is shown in Fig. 25(a). Once again the recovery with the classical SI is not acceptable. These two examples also demonstrate the need for a *known* reference pulse in the classical SI, to recover $g(t)$ from $C_{SI}(t)$.

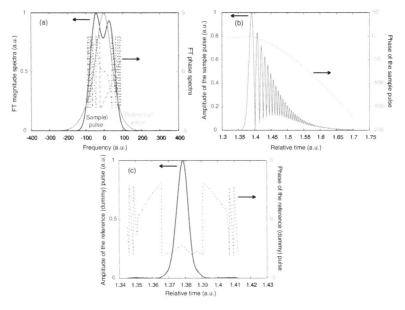

Fig. 24. (a)FT magnitude and phase spectrum of the reference and sample pulses; (b) temporal profile of the sample pulse; (c) temporal profile of the reference pulse.

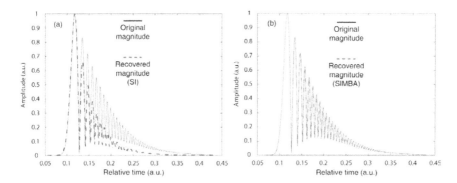

Fig. 25. Recovery results for the amplitude of the sample pulse using (a) classical SI; (b) SIMBA.

For the classical SI approach, (with or without a known reference pulse), as mentioned earlier, there is only one requirement: the bandwidth of the reference pulse, BW_f should roughly cover the bandwidth of the sample pulse, BW_g, i.e., $BW_f \geq\sim BW_g$. For SIMBA, the requirements, once again, can be summarized as:

(1) The same bandwidth requirement as in the classical SI, stated above, i.e., $BW_f \geq\sim BW_g$ is needed.

(2) $max\left\{f(t)\right\}$ should be greater than $max\left\{g(t)\right\}$ by at least 5-10 times.

(3) The temporal width of $f(t)$ should be narrower than the temporal width of $g(t)$, by $>\sim 5$ times.

Under these set of conditions, the classical SI approach still yields nothing more than $C_{SI}(t) = g(t) * f(t)$, which without the reference pulse information cannot yield a correct solution to the sample pulse $g(t)$. This is actually illustrated in Figs. 23 and 25, i.e., the reference and sample pulses shown in these examples have been chosen to satisfy the above-listed three requirements of SIMBA. The result of the classical SI (*without* the reference information) yields an unacceptable error for the recovery of the sample pulse, $g(t)$. However, for the same pulses shown in Figs. 22 and 24, SIMBA yields very good recovery under the above-mentioned set of conditions (see Figs. 23 and 25(b)). The error in the recovery is reduced by more than an order of magnitude using SIMBA. These

119

examples clearly demonstrate the outstanding performance of SIMBA with respect to the classical IFT based SI approach.

To better understand the observed differences between the classical SI and SIMBA, we should note that SIMBA heavily depends on the ratio between $max\{f(t)\}$ and $max\{g(t)\}$ as already shown in Fig. 12. In other words, the improvements obtained using SIMBA over the conventional SI require a ratio of $max\{f(t)\}/max\{g(t)\} >\sim 5-10$. However the classical SI approach does not depend on this ratio, i.e., exactly the same unacceptable recovery results of SI (e.g., see Fig. 25(a)) could have been obtained with a field ratio of e.g., 1. This observed difference between SI and SIMBA is primarily due to the fact that the MPF based iterative error-reduction algorithm retrieves the FT phase of $|S(f)|$ in order to recover at the end a *causal* MPF function, i.e., $s(t) = f(t) + g(t-\tau)$. However, with the classical SI, the recovered quantity is a non-causal function of time, i.e., it extends in both the negative and positive time domains (taking a direct IFT of Eq. (1) yields $IFT\{|S(f)|^2\} = IFT\{|F(f)|^2 + |G(f)|^2\} + C_{SI}(t-\tau) + \tilde{C}_{SI}(-t-\tau)$, where $\tilde{C}_{SI}$ stands for the complex conjugate of C_{SI}).

Furthermore, in the classical SI, in order to recover $C_{SI}(t-\tau)$, the delay parameter τ has to be chosen carefully such that it does not overlap in time with the term $IFT\{|F(f)|^2 + |G(f)|^2\}$. However, this temporal aliasing is not an issue for SIMBA since it directly recovers $s(t) = f(t) + g(t-\tau)$. This means that the choice of τ in SIMBA is not as critical as it is for SI. Another important advantage of SIMBA over the classical SI is that the signal-to-noise ratio is improved by a factor of two, since the former uses $|S(f)|$ whereas the latter uses $|S(f)|^2$.

5.5 EXPERIMENTAL RESULTS

In this section of the thesis, two different experimental demonstrations of SIMBA will be presented. Both of these experiments use a femtosecond laser as the dummy pulse to characterize an output (sample) pulse that results from the interaction of the dummy pulse with an optical system that is of interest (Fig. 26). In each case, the results of SIMBA will be compared to other conventional pulse characterization tools such as FROG or TADPOLE.

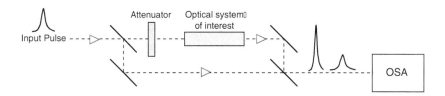

Fig. 26. General block diagram of the reported experiments.

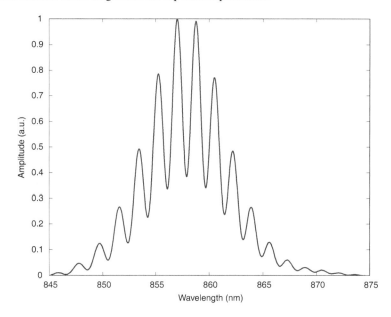

Fig. 27 Measured power spectrum corresponding to the pulse sequence of the material-characterization experiment of Ref. 10.

In the first experiment, the optical system of interest consisted of slab of fused silica (~16 cm long). Therefore, the experiment can be thought of as a material-characterization experiment. The input dummy pulse was ~145 fs long (FWHM), generated from a Ti:Sapphire oscillator that ran at ~859nm with a repetition rate of 96

MHz.[10] The peak powers of the dummy and sample pulses were 2.61 μW and 168 nW, respectively, which corresponds to a maximum field ratio of ~4.[10] Other details of the experiment can also be found in Ref. 10. The measured power spectrum of the pulse sequence formed by delaying the dummy pulse with respect to the sample pulse is shown in Fig. 27. Because of the fact that fused silica has a large transparency window with $\chi^{(2)}$ ≈ 0, the bandwidth of the sample pulse roughly matches that of the input dummy pulse. This is also visible in the recorded power spectrum (Fig. 27), i.e., the interference between the two pulses occurs all across the available bandwidth. The effect of the thick slab of fused silica is simply to broaden the dummy pulse by putting a strong second-order spectral phase, without affecting the bandwidth of the dummy pulse. The result of the recovery, after applying SIMBA to the square-root of the measured power spectrum (Fig. 27) is shown in Fig. 28. For comparison purposes, the results of the recovery obtained with both FROG and TADPOLE techniques are also shown.

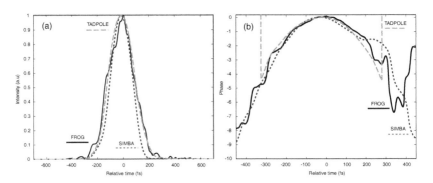

Fig. 28. Results of the recovery of the sample pulse (a) intensity, and (b) phase from the measured power spectrum shown in Fig. 27.

The general agreement in the recovery results, for both the intensity and phase of the electric field profile, obtained using SIMBA, FROG and TADPOLE is very good. Note that the recovery results of TADPOLE, which also relies on the measured power spectrum shown in Fig. 27, involved two additional measurements: an initial full characterization of the dummy pulse using a FROG set-up, and then an extra power spectrum measurement for the unknown sample pulse alone. However SIMBA only used the measured power spectrum shown in Fig. 27 for the recovery. Note also that in this experiment, the temporal width requirement of SIMBA is not fully satisfied: FWHM of the dummy pulse is only ~1.7 times narrower than the FWHM of the sample pulse. However, the recovery results obtained with SIMBA are still quite good. Especially, the spectral phase, shown in Fig. 28(b) agrees very well with other techniques and also with the predicted phase spectrum that can be theoretically computed using the known dispersion coefficients of fused silica.[10] Note also that for the spectral phase recovery, after a certain range, where the intensity of the pulse drops significantly, the recovered phase curves start to diverge from each other. This result is expected and inconsequential, as already discussed in earlier sections.

In the second experiment, the optical system of interest (Fig. 26) involved a thin film bandpass filter (FWHM ~ 10 nm) that significantly filtered the frequency bandwidth of the dummy pulse. This spectral filtering resulted in a temporally wider sample pulse, as required by SIMBA. In this experiment, the dummy pulse FWHM was ~30 fs. To test the repeatability of SIMBA, using the same set-up, two successive measurements were made with slightly different delay values between the sample and dummy pulses. The recorded CCD images at the OSA for each measurement are shown in Fig. 29. The resolution of the spectrum analyzer was ~54 pm. A maximum field ratio of ~4.40 and ~4.17 was used in Figs. 29(a) and 29(b), respectively, between the dummy and sample pulses.

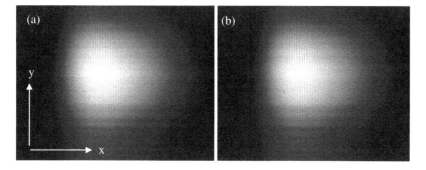

Fig. 29. Recorded CCD images corresponding to the power spectra measurement of the pulse sequence for the second experiment. The delay parameter together with the maximum field ratio between the sample and dummy pulses are different in (a) and (b).

Note that the recorded CCD images are two-dimensional. Since the complex electric field profile of the pulses are one-dimensional, in principle, only an array of CCD pixels could be used, for instance a single line along x direction (Fig. 29) would have been sufficient. However, to improve the signal-to-noise ratio in the measurement, a two-dimensional CCD array was preferred. By adding up all the recorded spatial FT magnitude spectra along y, we can get the measured power spectrum corresponding to the input pulse sequence for each case as shown in Figs. 30 (a) and (b), respectively.

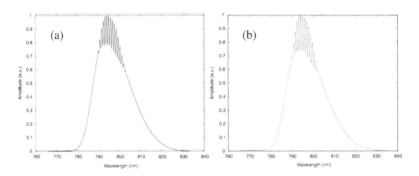

Fig. 30. The power spectrum computed by adding all the recorded spectra of Figs. 29(a) and (b), respectively, along y direction.

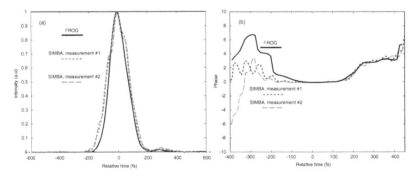

Fig. 31. The recovered intensity and phase of the sample pulse for the second experiment.

Comparing Figs. 27 and 30, one can realize that due to the presence of the bandpass filter in the second experiment, the bandwidth of the sample pulse is significantly reduced. This bandwidth reduction translates itself into the fact that the interference now occurs only at the center region of whole available bandwidth of the dummy pulse (see Fig. 30). Furthermore, the similarity between the simulation curves of Figs. 9(b) and 17(b) and the experimental curves of Fig. 30 is worth noting.

Applying SIMBA to the square-root of each of the power spectra shown in Figs. 30(a) and 30(b), the intensity and phase of the electric field of the sample pulse can be recovered as shown in Figs. 31(a) and 31(b), respectively. For comparison purposes the results of a commercial FROG set-up for the same sample pulse are also shown in Fig. 31. Once again the agreement between the results of SIMBA and FROG is quite good. It should be noted that the used FROG set-up was based on second-harmonic generation, and therefore had time reversal ambiguity in its results. The time reversal ambiguity of FROG results was corrected using SIMBA, such that Fig. 31(a) has the correct time axis. It is also noteworthy that both techniques reliably recovered the satellite pulse (with a smaller amplitude) between 200-400 fs (Fig. 31(a)). The physical origin of this satellite pulse is the spectral side lobes created by the bandpass filter used in the experiment. Once again, the observed discrepancy in the recovered phase spectra, especially for $t < \sim$-200 fs is simply due to a significant reduction in the pulse intensity.

The consistency between the two successive SIMBA measurements is also worth mentioning for the repeatability of SIMBA results with different delay and maximum field ratios. The mechanical stability of the used experimental set-up was much less than a micron, which directly means that the delay jitter in the experiment would be lower than 1 fs. Finally, in both of the reported experiments, the interferometric measurement systems were kept at room temperature, i.e., were far away from being shot-noise limited. However, this still enabled us to recover the sample pulse complex electric field profiles quite reliably.

5.6 CONCLUSIONS

We have introduced a different approach to spectral interferometry, SIMBA, a simple and yet powerful technique that can characterize weak ultra-short pulses. SIMBA involves forming a sequence consisting of a dummy pulse of *unknown* profile followed by the unknown sample pulse that need to be characterized. This sequence is then sent to a simple spectrum analyzer, the output of which is processed to recover both the phase and the magnitude of the sample pulse's electric field profile. If the reference pulse electric field amplitude is larger than the unknown pulse amplitude (e.g., by a factor of >5) and also if the reference pulse temporal width is narrower than the temporal width of the unknown sample pulse (e.g., by a factor of >5), then using a minimum phase based processing, the complex electric field of the sample pulse can be recovered *without the need for a known reference pulse*. Under these conditions, this recovery is unique. The first requirement of SIMBA, however, is quite loose, which actually is almost always satisfied in characterization of weak ultrashort pulses using stronger reference pulses. The second requirement, on the other hand, makes SIMBA especially suitable for characterization of highly chirped weak pulses such as in pump-probe experiments. In such cases, if need be, a linear pulse compressor can also be utilized to generate a narrower dummy pulse from the sample pulse itself. SIMBA shares all the benefits of SI such as being a linear technique that can characterize weak ultrashort pulses, having a simple measurement set-up (a single spectrum analyzer is used), having no time reversal ambiguity, etc. Furthermore there is no minimum constraint for the time delay between the reference and sample pulses, and multiple (identical or different) pulses can be simultaneously characterized using a single power spectrum measurement. This combination of features makes SIMBA an important tool to characterize weak ultra-short pulses in real time.

REFERENCES

1. Jean-Claude Diels and Wolfgang Rudolph, Ultrashort Laser Pulse Phenomena: Fundamentals, Techniques and Applications on a Femtosecond Time Scale, (Elsevier, Academic Press, London, 1996)

2. M. R. Hee, J. A. Izatt, E. A. Swanson, and J. G. Fujimoto, "Femtosecond transillumination tomography in thick tissue", Opt. Lett. 18, 1107, (1993)

3. X. Liu, D. Du; and G. Mourou, "Laser ablation and micromachining with ultrashort laser pulses", IEEE J. Quantum Electron. 33, 1706, (1997)

4. K. M. Davis, K. Miura, N. Sugimoto, and K. Hirao, "Writing waveguides in glass with a femtosecond laser" Opt. Lett. 21, 1729, (1996)

5. A. M. Weiner, J. P. Heritage, and J. A. Salehi, "Encoding and decoding of femtosecond pulses", Opt. Lett. 13, 300, (1988)

6. K. L. Sala, G. A. Kenney-Wallace, and G. E. Hall, "CW autocorrelation measurements of picosecond laser pulses", IEEE J. Quantum Electron. QE-16, 990, (1980)

7. J. L. A. Chilla and O. E. Martinez, "Direct determination of the amplitude and the phase of femtosecond light pulses", Opt. Lett. 16, 39, (1991)

8. R. Trebino, and D. J. Kane, "Using phase retrieval to measure the intensity and phase of ultrashort pulses: frequency-resolved optical gating", J. Opt. Soc. Am. A 10, 1101, (1993)

9. D. E. Tokunaga, A. Terasaki, and T. Kobayashi, "Femtosecond continuum interferometer for transient phase and transmission spectroscopy", J. Opt. Soc. Am. B 13, 496 (1996)

10. D. N. Fittinghoff, *et al.,* "Measurement of the intensity and phase of ultraweak, ultrashort laser pulses", Opt. Lett. 21, 884 (1996)

11. D. Meshulach, D. Yelin and Y. Silberberg, "Real-time spatial-spectral interference measurements of ultrashort optical pulses", J. Opt. Soc. Am. B 14, 2095 (1997)

12. C. Iaconis and I. A. Walmsley, "Spectral phase interferometry for direct electric-field reconstruction of ultrashort optical pulses", Opt. Lett. 23, 792 (1998)

13. J. Debeau, B. Kowalski and R. Boittin, "Simple method for the complete characterization of an optical pulse", Opt. Lett. 23 1784-1786 (1998)

14. P. Kockaert, J. Azana, L. R. Chen and S. LaRochelle, "Full characterization of uniform ultrahigh-speed trains of optical pulses using fiber Bragg gratings and linear detectors", IEEE Phot. Technol. Lett. 16, 1540-1542 (2004)

15. S. Linden, H. Giessen and J. Kuhl, "XFROG- A new method for amplitude and phase characterization of weak ultrashort pulses", Phys. Stat. Sol. (B) 206, 119 (1998)

16. J. Peatross and A. Rundquist, "Temporal decorrelation of short laser pulses", J. Opt. Soc. Am. B 15, 216 (1998)

17. J. W. Nicholson, J. Jasapara, W. Rudolph, F. G. Omenetto and A. J. Taylor, "Full-field characterization of femtosecond pulses by spectrum and cross-correlation measurements", Opt. Lett. 24, 1774 (1999)

18. J. Chung and A. M. Weiner, "Ambiguity of ultrashort pulse shapes retrieved from the intensity autocorrelation and the power spectrum", IEEE J. Select. Quantum Electron. 656 (2001)

19. V. Oppenheim and R. W. Schafer, *Digital Signal Processing*, (Prentice Hall, 2002), Chap. 7.

20. T. F. Quatieri, Jr., and A. V. Oppenheim, "Iterative techniques for minimum phase signal reconstruction from phase or magnitude," IEEE Trans. Acoust., Speech, Signal Processing 29, 1187 (1981)

21. M. Hayes, J. S. Lim, and A. V. Oppenheim, "Signal reconstruction from phase or magnitude," IEEE Trans. Acoust., Speech, Signal Processing 28, 672 (1980)

22. J. R. Fienup, "Reconstruction of an object from the modulus of its Fourier transform," Opt. Lett. 3, 27 (1978)

23. R. W. Gerchberg and W. O. Saxton, "Practical algorithm for the determination of phase from image and diffraction plane pictures," Optik 35, 237 (1972)

24. A. Ozcan, M. J. F. Digonnet, and G. S. Kino, "Iterative processing of second-order optical nonlinearity depth profiles," Opt. Express 12, 3367 (2004), http://www.opticsexpress.org/abstract.cfm?URI=OPEX-12-15-3367

25. A. Ozcan, M. J. F. Digonnet, and G. S. Kino, "Group delay recovery using iterative processing of amplitude of transmission spectra of fibre Bragg gratings," Electron. Lett. 40, 1104 (2004)

26. M. Nisoli, S. De Silvestri, and O. Svelto, "Generation of high energy 10 fs pulses by a new pulse compression technique", Appl. Phys. Lett. 68, 2793 (1996)

27. M. A. Arbore, A. Galvanauskas, D. Harter, M. H. Chou, and M. M. Fejer, "Engineerable compression of ultrashort pulses by use of second-harmonic generation in chirped-period-poled lithium niobate", Opt. Lett. 22, 1341 (1997)

28. M. M. Wefers and K. A. Nelson, "Analysis of programmable ultrashort waveform generation using liquid-crystal spatial light modulators", J. Opt. Soc. Am. B 12, 1343 (1995)

29. A. Rundquist, A.Efimov, and D. H. Reitze, "Pulse shaping with the Gerchberg-Saxton algorithm", J. Opt. Soc. Am. B 19, 2468 (2002)

CHAPTER 6: NON-INTERFEROMETRIC CHARACTERIZATION OF FIBER BRAGG GRATINGS BASED ON MINIMUM-PHASE FUNCTIONS

This chapter concerns the non-interferometric characterization of fiber Bragg gratings (FBGs) using minimum phase function concepts. Specifically, we report a powerful application of the iterative error-reduction algorithm, presented in earlier chapters, to recover the whole complex transmission spectrum of *any* FBG from *only* its group delay spectrum *or* magnitude spectrum. Both theoretical simulations and experiments confirm this non-interferometric approach to be quite simple, fast and accurate, which makes it well suited for the practical design of fiber Bragg gratings with desired spectral features. The non-interferometric techniques presented in this chapter are applicable to all transmission gratings, together with any uniform or symmetric reflection grating. The experimental FBG transmission spectra reported in this chapter were provided by David Pureur of Highwave Optical Technologies, Lannion, France. All the relevant data analysis together with the principles of theory were developed by Aydogan Ozcan under the supervision of Gordon S. Kino and Michel J. F. Digonnet.

6.1 INTRODUCTION

There are many important applications of fiber Bragg gratings (FBGs), especially in optical communications, sensors, and biology.[1-3] In all of these applications, the knowledge of the spectral properties of the FBG are crucial. In general, an FBG can be characterized by its complex reflection spectrum, $r(\omega) = |r(\omega)| \cdot exp(j\phi_r)$, or complex transmission spectrum, $t(\omega) = |t(\omega)| \cdot exp(j\phi_t)$, where ω is the angular frequency, ϕ_r and ϕ_t are the phases of $r(\omega)$ and $t(\omega)$, respectively. Some applications require a specific spectrum for $|r(\omega)|$ or $|t(\omega)|$. These two quantities are easy to measure. Other applications require a specific spectrum for the group delay (or phase) of $r(\omega)$ or $t(\omega)$. (The group delays in reflection and transmission are defined as $d\phi_r(\omega)/d\omega$ and $d\phi_t(\omega)/d\omega$, respectively.) Therefore, for characterization, it is quite important to know both the magnitude and the group delay spectra of an FBG. On the other hand, from a design point of view, in order to fabricate a target FBG that has the desired spectral properties, both $r(\omega)$ and $t(\omega)$ need to be known. For the fabrication process, the required refractive index modulation of the target FBG can be computed from the knowledge of $r(\omega)$ and $t(\omega)$ (Fig. 1) for example by various layer peeling algorithms.[1-2] However, $r(\omega)$ and $t(\omega)$ are not independent quantities. For a lossless grating $|r(\omega)|^2 + |t(\omega)|^2 = 1$, which implies that the information of $|t(\omega)|$ can be obtained from $|r(\omega)|$ or vice versa.

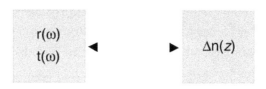

Fig. 1. The refractive index modulation of the FBG, $\Delta n(z)$, where z is the direction of light propagation in the fiber, can be uniquely recovered from the knowledge of $r(\omega)$ and $t(\omega)$. The other way is also possible: $r(\omega)$ and $t(\omega)$ can be uniquely recovered from the knowledge of $\Delta n(z)$.

  The purpose of this chapter is to introduce a simple and powerful technique that can relate the magnitude and group delay spectrum of FBGs to one another. We show, both through simulations and experimentally, that a simple and fast iterative error-reduction algorithm can be used to recover the whole complex transmission spectrum, $t(\omega)$, of any FBG (chirped, asymmetric, symmetric, uniform, etc.), using only the information of its group delay $(d\phi_t(\omega)/d\omega)$ *or* magnitude $(|t(\omega)|)$. Furthermore, if the FBG is known to be either symmetric *or* uniform, then the whole complex reflection spectrum, $r(\omega)$, can also be recovered from only the information of its group delay $(d\phi_r(\omega)/d\omega)$ *or* magnitude $(|r(\omega)|)$. In the first half of this chapter, the group delay spectrum is recovered from the magnitude spectrum measurement. This is a common situation encountered especially in testing commercial FBGs. Usually a direct measurement of the group delay spectrum requires a rather involved equipment such as an optical network analyzer. The powerful iterative approach presented in the first half of this chapter provides an elegant simpler solution to this problem. The second half of this chapter, which involves the recovery of the magnitude spectrum from a given group delay spectrum, is mostly helpful for the design of FBGs rather than their testing. The reason is that the measurement of group delay spectrum is much more complicated than the measurement of magnitude spectrum, and any equipment that can measure the group delay spectrum can also naturally measure the magnitude spectrum. However, in the design process of FBGs, it is desirable to retrieve the magnitude spectrum associated with a target group delay spectrum.

We believe that the results of this chapter are especially important for the design, fabrication and testing of FBGs with desired spectral features. Furthermore, because we anticipate that our technique will also be quite useful to establish the correlation between the imperfections (e.g., ripples) in the magnitude spectrum and the imperfections in the phase spectrum of an FBG, it can also be used to improve the fabrication process of practical FBGs.

6.2 ITERATIVE ERROR-REDUCTION ALGORITHM AND ITS APPLICATION TO FBG'S

In this section, the application of iterative error-reduction algorithms such as the Fienup algorithm [4] or the Gerchberg-Saxton algorithm [5] will be presented for two significant problems related to FBGs: (1) group delay recovery from magnitude spectrum, and (2) magnitude spectrum recovery from group delay spectrum.

6.2.1 GROUP DELAY RECOVERY FROM THE MAGNITUDE SPECTRUM

As mentioned in the introduction, measuring the full complex spectrum (e.g., $|t(\omega)|$ and $\phi_t(\omega)$) of an FBG is very important for almost all applications utilizing this technology. To this end, interferometric measurement systems such as optical coherence-domain reflectometry[6], Michelson interferometers[7] or end-reflection interference[8], can be used. However, interferometric measurement systems are in general relatively complex and exhibit a strong sensitivity to measurement noise. In contrast, measuring the magnitude spectrum of an FBG, e.g., $|t(\omega)|$ or $|r(\omega)|$, is much simpler and less sensitive to noise. However, a fundamental limitation of a simple magnitude measurement is that it does not provide the required phase information, $\phi_r(\omega)$ or $\phi_t(\omega)$.

From a user point of view, while an interferometric measurement tool, such as an optical network analyzer, is a costly piece of test equipment that is seldom available on a photo-writing set-up, an amplitude measurement system is always installed in such a system. Phase spectrum determination from amplitude measurement is therefore an economic, simple and fast approach to fully characterize FBGs.

Different methods have already been proposed to recover the missing phase or group delay information using only the measurement of $|r(\omega)|$ or $|t(\omega)|$.[9-13] To summarize, the reconstruction technique presented in Ref. 9 works only for uniform gratings, and it has been independently shown not to be suited for gratings with imperfections.[10] A similar technique[11] has been offered to improve the noise performance of the initial technique[9]. However, it is still limited to only uniform gratings, and the processing algorithm requires adjusting filtering parameters, which change from one FBG to the other.[11] One of the most promising efforts to recover the phase information from the amplitude spectrum of FBGs is the work of Poladian.[12] His technique utilizes the fact that the transmission spectra of *all* FBGs belong to the family of minimum phase functions (MPF), i.e., their phase and magnitude are related by the complex Hilbert transform. In Poladian's technique, the transmission group delay of FBGs is recovered by applying the Hilbert transformation to the measured spectrum of $|t(\omega)|$. His technique works very well, but the numerical evaluation of the Hilbert transform integral is not trivial, and is rather noise sensitive.[9,12]

In our recent work,[13] we proposed a simpler, faster and less noise sensitive technique that exploits the same MPF property and also works for *any* FBG (chirped, asymmetric, symmetric, uniform, etc.), but that is based on the application of the iterative error reduction algorithm discussed in Chapter 2. Our technique can recover the transmission group delay of *any* FBG from only the measured transmission spectrum $|t(\omega)|$. Furthermore, if the FBG is known to be symmetric or uniform, the reflection group delay of the FBG can also be uniquely determined by this technique. The fundamental difference between Poladian's work and our approach is that our technique relies on a simpler and less noise sensitive iterative approach.

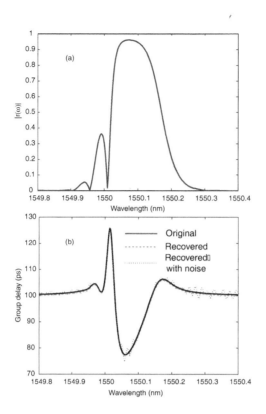

Fig. 2. (a) Magnitude of the reflection spectrum of an arbitrarily chosen Gaussian-apodized symmetric grating. (b) Group delay of this grating as a function of wavelength. The solid black curve is the theoretical group delay; the dashed gray curve is the group delay recovered by the Fienup algorithm (100 iterations). The dotted light gray curve is the recovered group delay when a 5% uniform noise is added to the square of the transmission spectrum amplitude.

Implementation of the iterative error reduction algorithm to recover the group delay of an FBG from its measured magnitude spectrum is the same as discussed in Chapter 5. Instead of the complex electric field envelope function $e(t)$ of Chapter 5, this time we deal with the complex impulse response of the FBG, $h_T(t)$, where $h_T(t)$ is simply the IFT of $t(\omega)$. More discussion will be presented on the concept of impulse response of FBGs in the second half of this chapter. The data that is fed into the algorithm is the measured magnitude of the transmission spectrum of the FBG, labeled $|t_M(\omega)|$.

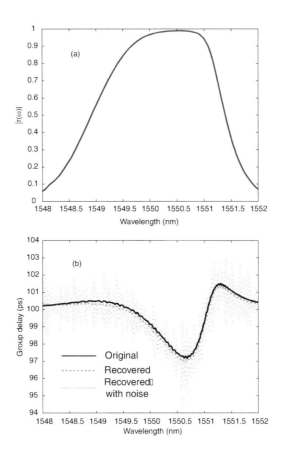

Fig. 3. Same as Fig. 2, except the FBG is asymmetric and chirped.

For a lossless grating, $|t_M(\omega)|$ can be obtained from the measurement of the magnitude of the FBG's reflection spectrum, labeled $|r_M(\omega)|$, which satisfies $|t_M(\omega)|^2 + |r_M(\omega)|^2 = 1$. At the end of the nth iteration, $\phi_n(\omega)$ is the recovered transmission phase spectrum of the FBG. The group delay is then simply calculated as the derivative of the phase, $d\phi_n(\omega)/d\omega$. Since it has been empirically shown that the error reduction loop converges to the MPF corresponding to a given FT magnitude,[14,15] the fact that the transmission spectrum of any FBG is *always* an MPF ensures the convergence of our technique to the unique phase spectrum, so that $\phi_n(\omega) \to \phi_t(\omega)$.

6.2.1.1 Simulation results

To verify the validity of our approach, we applied the Fienup algorithm to the transmission spectrum magnitude of various FBGs. Figures 2 and 3 display two arbitrarily chosen examples tested in these simulations: a symmetric Gaussian-apodized grating (Fig. 2) and a non-symmetric chirped grating (Fig. 3). The magnitude of the reflection spectrum of each grating is shown in Figs. 2(a) and 3(a), respectively. In Figs. 2(b) and 3(b), the theoretical transmission group delay, which is computed using the transfer matrix formalism developed in Ref. 3, is shown as solid black curves, and the group delay (without any noise present) recovered by the Fienup algorithm is shown as dashed gray curves. These simulations required $n = 100$ iterations and took only a few seconds on a 500-MHz computer. For each FBG, the recovered group delay curve is very close to the original curve. In each case, the curves have essentially the same shape except for an average dc offset of the order of ~0.1-0.2 ps. This phenomenon is not specific to our technique; similar dc offsets are also observed with other techniques.[9,11,12]

To demonstrate the noise performance of the algorithm, each theoretical $|t(\omega)|^2$ spectrum was multiplied by a uniform noise with a mean of 1 and an amplitude of 5%; the Fienup algorithm was then applied to these noisy spectra. The group delays recovered, again after 100 iterations in each case, are shown as the light gray dotted curves in Figs. 2(b) and 3(b). Once again, in each case, the recovery is very good, which demonstrates the usefulness and robustness of the proposed algorithm, even in the presence of fairly strong noise.

6.2.1.2 Experimental results

To experimentally verify this powerful technique, we applied it to a 72 mm long chirped dispersion compensator FBG. The effective index (n_{eff}) of this FBG for LP_{01} mode is 1.447. The measured transmission magnitude of this FBG is shown in Fig. 4. The high frequency ripples observed in Fig. 4 are due to imperfections arising primarily from multiple interferences inside the grating during the UV writing process.[16] For comparison purposes, the group delay spectrum of the same FBG was also measured using a commercial phase shift set-up (Advantest Q7760) with a 250 MHz modulation frequency, a 3-pm resolution and using the high sensitivity mode (Fig. 5). Applying the iterative Fienup loop as described Chapter 5 to the measured transmission spectrum of Fig. 4, after $n = 100$ iterations, which took a few sec using a 500 MHz computer, produced the group delay spectrum of the FBG as shown in Fig. 5. As can be seen, the recovered group delay spectrum agrees very well with the measured group delay spectrum. This near-perfect agreement demonstrates the robustness, accuracy and convenience of this powerful technique.

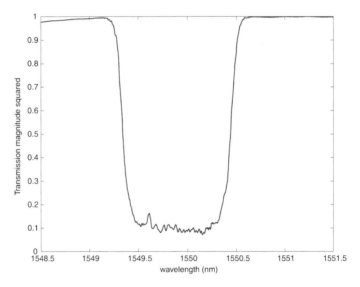

Fig. 4. Measured transmission magnitude squared for the chirped dispersion compensator FBG module. Total length of this chirped FBG is 72 mm with an effective index of 1.447.

Application of this technique to other practical FBGs, such as a broadband gain flattening FBG operating across ~40 nm, between ~1527 nm and ~1567 nm, produced similar results with very good group delay recovery across the whole spectrum. The measured magnitude of the transmission spectrum of this chirped gain flattening FBG, with a total length of $L = 14.5$ mm and $n_{eff} = 1.448$, is shown in Fig. 6. The result of the recovery for this FBG is shown in Fig. 7. To better appreciate the details of this recovered spectrum, several sample windows (with a period of ~10 nm) across the operation bandwidth of the device are shown in Figs. 7(a)-(d). Once again, the results are quite good.

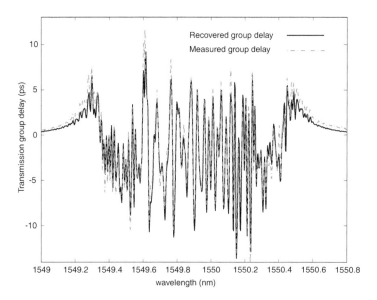

Fig. 5. Measured (dashed curve) and recovered (solid curve) group delay spectra of the chirped dispersion compensator FBG module.

Figures 5 and 7 demonstrate that our iterative approach works quite well for both narrowband and broadband FBGs, which stresses its versatility. The experimental results also reveal that our technique can be conveniently used as a monitor for imperfections in the grating writing process. In other words, this technique can be used as a tool to understand which parts of the imperfections in the amplitude spectrum cause the unwanted ripples in the group delay spectrum. Establishing this correlation is an important step towards improving the fabrication process of FBGs. Appendix D further illuminates this issue by outlining an *analytical* treatment of the relationship between the unwanted ripples in the amplitude spectrum and the observed ripples in the group delay spectrum of any FBG.

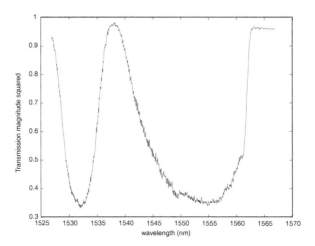

Fig. 6. Measured transmission magnitude squared for the broadband (~40 nm) gain flattening FBG module. Total length of this chirped FBG is 14.5 mm with an effective index of 1.448.

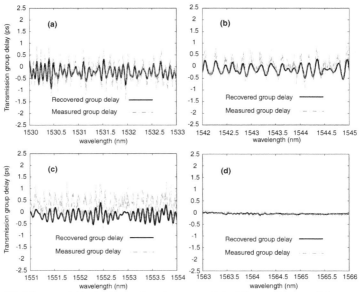

Fig. 7(a)-(d). Measured (dashed curve) and recovered (solid curve) group delay spectra of the gain flattening FBG module. To see the results of the recovery better, 4 different wavelength windows are shown in (a)-(d).

In the previous section, we applied the iterative error reduction algorithm to recover the group delay spectrum of an FBG from its measured magnitude spectrum. The experimental results proved that our technique works very well, and is quite robust to experimental noise. In this section, we will concentrate on the reverse the problem, which is useful for the design of FBGs: computing the magnitude spectrum of an FBG given its group delay spectrum.

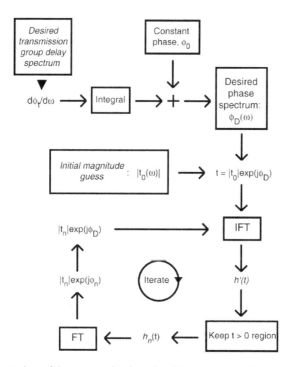

Fig. 8. Implementation of the error reduction algorithm to recover the magnitude spectrum corresponding to a desired group delay spectrum.

Retrieving the magnitude spectrum corresponding to a given group delay curve is not an issue in testing and characterization of FBGs. The reason is that measuring the magnitude spectrum of an FBG is much simpler than measuring its group delay spectrum. Furthermore, any advanced equipment that can measure the group delay spectrum of an FBG can at the same time measure the magnitude spectrum rather easily. Therefore, this task of computing the magnitude spectrum for a given group delay spectrum may not appear to be very interesting. However, in most practical applications involving designing FBGs, a specific group delay (or phase) spectrum is desired. The functional form and features of the required group delay vary significantly from one application to another. Meanwhile, for fabrication, the magnitude information is also needed for a unique representation of the index modulation required for the grating writing process. Therefore, depending on the application, one needs not only the desired group delay spectrum but also the corresponding magnitude spectrum to fully characterize the properties of the FBG that will be written. Therefore, the results of this section should be quite useful for the design of FBGs with different group delay features. Such a complete characterization method located in the manufacturing set-up should permit a post-photowriting step while maintaining the coherence between the UV fringes and the already-written grating. Real time correction of the grating response (like UV trimming) can then be performed.

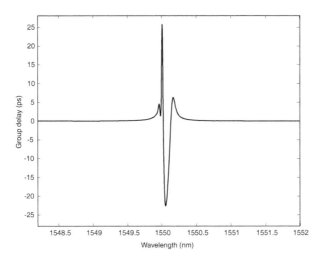

Fig. 9. Theoretical group delay spectrum of a Gaussian-apodised symmetric FBG. This is the only piece of information used to recover the magnitude of the transmission spectrum of the FBG.

The main difference from the previous section is that the targeted transmission phase spectrum is now known, but the transmission amplitude spectrum that will produce this phase spectrum is unknown. This problem can be solved by using the same basic principle of the error reduction algorithm, except that now the roles of the phase and the magnitude are reversed. Its implementation to recover the necessary magnitude of $t(\omega)$ given a desired group delay spectrum is shown in Fig. 8. Note once again that if the FBG is known to be symmetric or uniform, this same algorithm can be used to determine the magnitude of the *reflection* spectrum uniquely from its group delay.

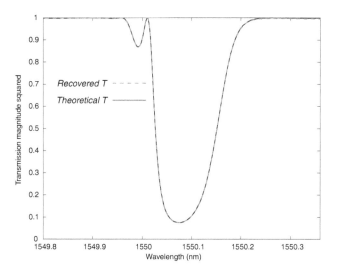

Fig. 10. The theoretical (solid line) and the recovered (dashed line) magnitude spectra of the same Gaussian-apodised symmetric FBG.

In Fig. 8, given a desired transmission group delay spectrum, $d\phi_t/d\omega$, the first step is to take the integral of the group delay to calculate the desired transmission phase spectrum, $\phi_D(\omega)$ for the FBG. It has been empirically established that the integration constant, ϕ_0, affects neither the convergence nor the result of the algorithm. Therefore, this constant can conveniently be chosen to be 0 or π for any FBG design. Furthermore, for cases where the desired transmission phase spectrum, $\phi_D(\omega)$ is known, the above-noted process of integration can conveniently be avoided. Once $\phi_D(\omega)$ has been computed or given, an initial guess for the missing magnitude spectrum is made, i.e., $|t_0(\omega)|$. As before, the convergence of the recovery algorithm is not affected by the choice of this initial guess, unless of course, $|t_0(\omega)| \approx 0$ is chosen, for which the algorithm can never converge. Therefore, the initial guess can be conveniently set at $|t_0(\omega)| = 1/2$. Since we have a first guess for the complex transmission spectrum, $t(\omega)$, we can start the iterations. The iteration loop in Fig. 8 is identical to the iteration given in Chapter 5, except for the final step. In the final step, rather than replacing the magnitude spectrum, the phase spectrum, ϕ_n, is now replaced with the desired phase spectrum $\phi_D(\omega)$, while maintaining the same magnitude spectrum, $|t_n|$ for the next iteration.

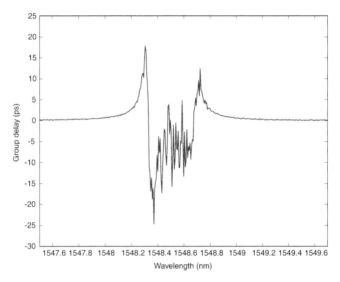

Fig. 11. Measured group delay spectrum of a chirped dispersion compensator FBG module. This is the only piece of information used to recover the magnitude of the transmission spectrum of the same FBG.

6.2.2.1 Simulation results

We first demonstrate the success of this technique with a numerical example, then proceed to experimental results in the next subsection. We have tested our technique on a Gaussian-apodised symmetric FBG. The theoretical group delay of this FBG, shown in Fig. 9, was computed using the piecewise-uniform transfer matrix approach of Ref. 3. Applying our algorithm (Fig. 8) to the group delay spectrum shown in Fig. 9, after $n = 100$ iterations, the magnitude of the transmission spectrum for the same FBG was recovered, as shown in Fig. 10. For comparison purposes, the theoretical magnitude spectrum of the same FBG (computed using the transfer matrix approach of Ref. 3) is also shown in Fig. 10. As can be seen, the magnitude recovery is excellent, with an error of less than 5 x 10^{-4} %, where the error is defined the same way as in Chapter 5. This result clearly demonstrates the power and accuracy of our technique.

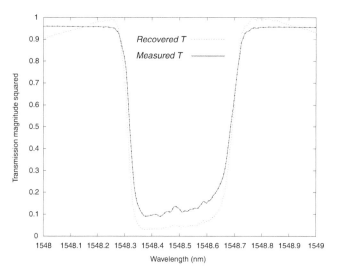

Fig. 12. The measured (solid line) and the recovered (dotted line) magnitude spectra of the same chirped dispersion compensator FBG module as in Fig. 11.

6.2.2.2 Experimental results

To evaluate our technique experimentally, we applied it to a chirped dispersion compensator FBG module. The group delay spectrum of this FBG module, shown in Fig. 11, was measured using the same Advantest instrument (250 MHz modulation frequency, 6 pm resolution). Applying our iterative technique, after $n = 100$ iterations, we recovered the magnitude spectrum as shown in Fig. 12. Once again, for comparison purposes, the measured transmission magnitude of the same FBG is also shown in Fig. 12. The magnitude recovery is very good, especially in the operation band of the FBG module, i.e., the useful band between ~1548.3 nm and ~1548.7 nm, where the notch occurs. In this wavelength range, the recovered magnitude curve has exactly the same fine features, e.g., ripples, as in the measured magnitude curve. The DC offset between the recovered and measured curves, especially at the notch position, is partly due to normalization errors that occurred during the measurement of the transmission magnitude of the FBG module. On the other hand, the discrepancy in the recovered profile, especially towards the edges of the measurement window, is due to the extra lengths of fiber pigtails used for testing on each side of the FBG. This additional length of fiber adds an artificial group delay to the measured transmission group delay curve. Although the length (~2.5 m each) and dispersion parameter (~17 ps/nm/km) of these fiber pigtails are known, and for normalization purposes, a total slope of 5m x 17ps/nm/km = 0.085ps/nm has been subtracted from the *initial* measured group delay spectrum (not shown), this phenomenon still adds experimental error to the slope of the group delay spectrum shown in Fig. 11. We believe that this additional slope error in the measured group delay curve is one of the main causes for the discrepancies observed in the recovered magnitude spectrum of Fig. 12, especially toward the ends of the measurement window. However, we also believe that this error does *not* constitute a fundamental limitation for our technique; for design purposes, the desired group delay (or phase) spectrum computation will be free of this source of error, in which case the recovery will be close to perfect, with an error of less than 5×10^{-4} %, as shown in Fig. 10.

6.3 CONCLUSIONS

In this chapter, we reported an important application of the iterative error-reduction algorithm to recover the entire complex spectrum of any transmission FBG, using only the information of its group delay *or* magnitude spectrum. The first half of the chapter dealt with the problem of retrieving the group delay spectrum of any transmission FBG from only its magnitude spectrum. Both simulation and experimental results confirmed our non-interferometric iterative approach to be quite simple, fast and accurate, making it especially suitable for testing commercial transmission FBGs. In the second half of this chapter, we dealt with the reverse problem, i.e., retrieving the magnitude spectrum given a transmission group delay curve. This problem, though hardly ever faced in testing FBGs, is especially suitable for the practical *design* and *fabrication* of FBGs with desired spectral features. It allows the designer to recover the unique transmission magnitude spectrum corresponding to the targeted group delay curve. This recovered information can then be used in conjunction with other design tools to fabricate the desired FBG. For this reverse problem, again both simulation and experimental results confirm that our technique is highly accurate.

REFERENCES

1. A. Othonos and K. Kalli, Fiber Bragg gratings: fundamentals and applications in telecommunications and sensing, (Artech House, Boston, 1999)

2. R. Kashyap, *Fiber Bragg Gratings*, (Academic Press, San Diego, 1999)

3. T. Erdogan, "Fiber grating spectra," J. Lightwave Technol. 15, 1277 (1997)

4. J. R. Fienup, "Reconstruction of an object from the modulus of its Fourier transform," Opt. Lett. 3, 27 (1978)

5. R. W. Gerchberg and W. O. Saxton, "Practical algorithm for the determination of phase from image and diffraction plane pictures," Optik 35, 237 (1972)

6. P. Lambelet, P. Y. Fonjallaz, H. G. Limberger, R. P. Salathe, C. H. Zimmer, and H. H. Gilgen, "Bragg grating characterization by optical low-coherence reflectometry," IEEE Photon. Technol. Lett. 5, 565 (1993)

7. D. W. Huang and C. C. Yang, "Reconstruction of fiber grating refractive-index profiles from complex Bragg reflection spectra," Appl. Opt. 38, 4494 (1999)

8. J. Skaar, "Measuring the group delay of fiber Bragg gratings by use of end-reflection interference," Opt. Lett. 24, 1020 (1999)

9. M. A. Muriel and A. Carballar, "Phase reconstruction from reflectivity in uniform fiber Bragg gratings," Opt. Lett. 22, 93 (1997)

10. J. Skaar and H. E. Engan, "Phase reconstruction from reflectivity in fiber Bragg gratings," Opt. Lett. 24, 136 (1999)

11. K. B. Rochford and S. D. Dyer, "Reconstruction of minimum-phase group delay from fibre Bragg grating transmittance/reflectance measurements," Electron. Lett. 35, 838 (1999)

12. L. Poladian, "Group-delay reconstruction for fiber Bragg gratings in reflection and transmission", Opt. Lett. 22, 1571 (1997)

13. A. Ozcan, M. J. F. Digonnet, and G. S. Kino, "Group delay recovery using iterative processing of amplitude of transmission spectra of fibre Bragg gratings," Electron. Lett. 40, 1104 (2004)

14. T. F. JR. Quatieri and A. V. Oppenheim, "Iterative techniques for minimum phase signal reconstruction from phase or magnitude," IEEE Transactions on Acoustics, Speech, and Signal Processing 29, 1187 (1981)

15. A. Ozcan, M. J. F. Digonnet, and G. S. Kino, "Iterative processing of second-order optical nonlinearity depth profiles," Opt. Express 12, 3367 (2004), http://www.opticsexpress.org/abstract.cfm?URI=OPEX-12-15-3367

16. M. Derrien, D. Gauden, E. Goyat, A. Mugnier, P. Yvernault, and D. Pureur, "Wavelength-frequency analysis of dispersion compensator group delay ripples," Optical Fiber Communication Conference, paper MF 31 (2003)

CHAPTER 7: INTERFEROMETRIC CHARACTERIZATION OF FIBER BRAGG GRATINGS BASED ON SIMBA

This chapter is concerned with the interferometric characterization of fiber Bragg gratings (FBGs) using minimum phase function concepts. The important advantage of this interferometric approach, which relies on Spectral Interferometry using Minimum-phase Based Algorithms (SIMBA), is that it can characterize both the reflection and transmission spectra of *any* FBG, without exceptions. The non-interferometric technique described in the previous chapter was limited to transmission FBGs and to symmetric or uniform reflection FBGs. Another important difference between this chapter and the previous one is that the aim of this chapter is to test (or characterize) both the magnitude and group delay spectra of FBGs using a single measurement, whereas Chapter 6 dealt with the problem of relating a given magnitude spectrum to its corresponding group delay spectrum or vice versa.

7.1 INTRODUCTION

The focus of this chapter will be interferometric systems utilizing Spectral Interferometry using Minimum-phase Based Algorithms (SIMBA) to fully characterize *any* fiber Bragg grating (FBG) spectra. The core of our approach involves sending an unknown dummy short laser pulse, e.g., ~1-30 ps of temporal width, into the FBG of interest, and using an optical spectrum analyzer (OSA) to record the spectrum of the interference between the reflected pulse from the grating and the time delayed version of the original short pulse. This measured spectrum, which yields the square of the Fourier transform (FT) magnitude of the input pulse sequence's electric field envelope, is then processed to uniquely recover both the phase and amplitude of the FBG spectrum. The underlying principle for this unique recovery is that by construction, the input pulse sequence sent to the OSA is close to a minimum phase function (MPF); thus, it is possible to recover its FT phase spectrum using only the knowledge of its FT magnitude spectrum. This is an important result since by merely measuring an FT magnitude, with a rather simple set-up the entire complex spectrum of the grating can be recovered. Furthermore, this technique can conveniently be used to simultaneously characterize more than one FBG, using a single FT magnitude measurement. This technique has significant advantages over existing techniques: a higher resolution, better noise performance and the ability to use longer duration laser pulses.

In principle, both the phase and the magnitude of an FBG spectrum [1-3] can be measured separately. The magnitude measurement is relatively simple compared to the phase spectrum measurement. Furthermore, as discussed in Chapter 6, for transmission gratings and for uniform or symmetric reflection gratings the phase spectrum (or the group delay spectrum) can be uniquely derived from the measured magnitude spectrum.[4,5] However, in general, for *an arbitrary* FBG the *direct* phase spectrum measurement is more complicated since it requires an interferometric set-up. In the Michelson interferometer approach,[6] which uses a tunable laser and an optical spectrum analyzer (OSA), the phase of the complex reflection spectrum is recovered from *three* independent measurements. In the end-reflection interferometry technique,[7] the FBG is again characterized using a tunable laser together with an OSA, by measuring the spectral reflectivity that is caused by the interference between the grating itself and the bare fiber end. This last technique, however, is destructive in that it requires the bare fiber end to be only a few cm away from the grating.

Among other interferometric techniques that can be used to fully characterize FBGs, low-coherence *time* reflectometry [8-11] is one of the most promising. It consists of a Michelson interferometer illuminated with a broadband light source. The light reflected both from the FBG of interest, placed in one arm of the interferometer, and from a moveable mirror placed in the reference arm, are coupled together and directed to the detector. A disadvantage is that this approach requires a slow mechanical scan to retrieve the impulse response of the FBG as a function of time. To avoid this slow scanning process, a low-coherence *spectral* interferometry set-up, which uses a pulsed laser source, has been recently suggested.[12,13] In this approach, a broadband laser pulse is sent to the FBG of interest, and the reflected pulse from the grating is temporally combined with a delayed replica of the input laser pulse. Next, this pulse sequence is sent to an OSA, which records its power spectrum. The constraint on the success of this technique is that the *autocorrelation* function of the pulsed laser must be temporally much narrower than the impulse response of the FBG, ideally like a delta function. In other words, the recovery of the impulse response of a given FBG is limited in resolution to the autocorrelation trace of the input laser pulse. Furthermore, the delay between the reflected pulse from the FBG and the input laser pulse must be carefully adjusted to avoid overlap in the inverse FT domain, which would make the recovery impossible due to aliasing.

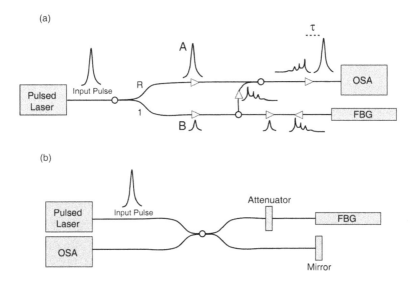

Fig. 1. (a) First proposed experimental set-up for full characterization of FBGs using SIMBA, (b) an alternative set-up that can be used for the same purpose.

This chapter introduces two different techniques utilizing SIMBA to retrieve both the phase and magnitude spectrum of an FBG from a single power spectrum measurement. The SIMBA technique was first used in Chapter 5 for the characterization of weak ultrashort pulses. In this chapter, we apply the basics of SIMBA to characterize FBGs, using the same two components required for the low-coherence *spectral* interferometry set-up already described, i.e., a pulsed input laser and an OSA. Our technique can be divided into two approaches. The experimental set-ups required for these two approaches are slightly different; the processing of the measured quantities for the characterization of the FBG, together with the principle of operation, are exactly identical.

In the first approach (Fig. 1), the laser pulse is first attenuated in power, either by an uneven beam splitter with a splitting ratio of R, where R > 1 (Fig. 1(a)), or by an attenuator (Fig. 1(b)). This pulse (labeled B in Fig. 1(a)) is then sent to the FBG of interest. Next, the reflected pulse from the FBG is temporally combined with the delayed unattenuated version of the input laser pulse (labeled A in Fig. 1(a)), to form a pulse sequence. This pulse sequence has a sharp peak at the leading edge, due to the unattenuated laser pulse, followed by the broader and much weaker pulse, reflected by the FBG. The key element, as discussed in Chapter 5, is that because of this feature, by construction this pulse sequence is close to an MPF, which makes it possible to recover its FT phase from only the measurement of its FT magnitude.[14] This formed pulse sequence is sent to an OSA, which yields the power spectrum or the square of the FT magnitude of the electric field envelope of the sequence. The measured power spectrum is then processed either analytically or iteratively to yield both the phase and magnitude spectra of the initial FBG.

This first approach offers important advantages over existing techniques, especially low-coherence *spectral* interferometry. First, with SIMBA, the delay between the reflected pulse and the laser pulse can be chosen arbitrarily small, as long as the two pulses temporally do not overlap. This choice is especially important because it enables the use of a lower resolution OSA, since the shorter the time delay between the two pulses, the lower the maximum frequency of oscillations in the power spectrum. A second advantage of the first approach is that it allows characterization of more than one FBG at the same time, using a single OSA measurement. Third, the processing involved in SIMBA is more robust to experimental noise, especially when compared with the processing involved in low-coherence *spectral* interferometry. Finally, with this first approach, the temporal width of the laser pulse must be significantly narrower than the impulse response of the FBG of interest. However, this requirement constitutes an improved constraint when compared with low-coherence *spectral* interferometry,[12,13] since the latter requires the *autocorrelation* function of the pulsed laser to be temporally much narrower than the impulse response of the grating. In other words, for the same FBG, SIMBA will yield roughly two times better resolution than low-coherence *spectral* interferometry.

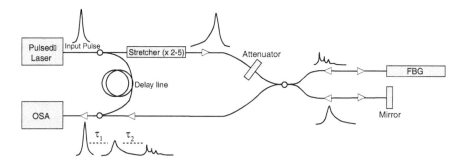

Fig. 2. Second proposed experimental set-up for full characterization of FBGs using SIMBA.

The second proposed approach utilizing SIMBA (Fig. 2) offers even more significant advantages over current approaches. Most importantly, the input laser pulse does not need to be temporally much narrower than the impulse response of the grating. To illustrate, low-coherence *spectral* interferometry requires for instance 1 ps laser source to accurately characterize an FBG with an impulse response of 100 ps duration. In comparison, our second approach only requires a ~50 ps laser pulse for the same FBG. In this second approach, shown in Fig. 2, a pulsed laser source with for instance a 50-ps temporal width is split into two pulses, one of which is sent to a delay line, while the other pulse is sent to a pulse stretcher, which broadens its temporal width by a factor of at least ~2-5. In practice, this pulse stretcher can simply be a loop of fiber optic cable. Next, this broadened pulse is sent through an attenuator, and then split into two weak pulses, as shown in Fig. 2. The reflections from the FBG of interest and from a reference mirror, which could in principle be a bare fiber end, are then temporally combined with the time-delayed version of the unattenuated initial laser pulse in the lower arm of the set-up, as shown in Fig. 2. This pulse sequence, which has a dominant pulse at the leading edge followed by two weaker reflected pulses, is then sent to an OSA to measure its power spectrum. The processing of the measured FT magnitude from the OSA and the principles of the recovery algorithm are identical to the approach of Fig. 1. Apart from the fact that it does not require a short laser pulse, this second approach also has all the benefits of the first approach. The only minor disadvantage of the second approach is that its experimental set-up is slightly more involved than either the first approach (Fig. 1) or low-coherence *spectral* interferometry.

Application of SIMBA to FBG characterization, as outlined above, relies on a particular property of minimum phase functions (MPFs) that allows one to relate the FT phase of the function to its FT magnitude either analytically or iteratively.[14-17] To our knowledge, this is the first time that this concept of MPFs has been applied to fully characterize any FBG spectra (transmission *or* reflection).

7.2 CONCEPT OF IMPULSE RESPONSE OF AN FBG AND MINIMUM PHASE FUNCTIONS

Mathematically, the transmission and reflection impulse response of an FBG, $h_T(t)$ and $h_R(t)$, where t is the relative time, are the inverse FTs of the complex field transmission and reflection spectra, $t(\omega)$ and $r(\omega)$, respectively, where ω is the angular frequency. Therefore, knowing the impulse response of an FBG means knowing the complex spectrum of the same grating as well. Because it is a complex quantity, the impulse response of an FBG is as challenging to measure as the whole complex spectrum of the grating.

It is well-known that the transmission impulse response of all FBGs belongs to the class of minimum phase functions (MPFs).[4,18] This enables retrieval of the whole complex transmission spectrum, $t(\omega)$, from only the measurement of its magnitude spectrum (reflection or transmission, since for a lossless grating $|t(\omega)|^2 + |r(\omega)|^2 = 1$). The recovery can conveniently be achieved by either analytical or iterative techniques.[4,5] The details of the iterative approach were discussed in Chapter 6. Unfortunately the reflection impulse response, $h_R(t)$, of an FBG is generally not an MPF, making it impossible to uniquely recover the whole complex reflection spectrum, $r(\omega)$, from only the magnitude spectrum measurement. However, once $|r(\omega)|$ has been characterized by some means, it directly implies that $t(\omega)$ is also fully characterized since $|t(\omega)|^2 = 1 - |r(\omega)|^2$ is now known.

7.3 CHARACTERIZATION OF FBG'S USING SIMBA

In this section, we discuss the application of SIMBA as a convenient tool to uniquely characterize the whole complex reflection and hence transmission spectra of all FBGs by recovering the reflection impulse response, $h_R(t)$, using a single FT magnitude measurement. As discussed in Chapter 5, the fundamental concept of SIMBA relies on the fact that by placing a strong pulse at the leading edge of a sequence of pulses, the whole pulse sequence, even if a complex quantity, becomes close to an MPF, which makes it possible to recover the phase information from only the FT magnitude measurements.

7.3.1 THE FIRST PROPOSED SIMBA SET-UP FOR FBG CHARACTERIZATION

Let us first describe step-by-step how the first proposed set-up (Fig. 1) actually works. By sending a short laser pulse, with a complex electric field envelope of $E(t)$, to an FBG, the reflected pulse spectrum can simply be calculated as $E_{Refl}(\omega) = E(\omega) \cdot r(\omega)$, where $E(\omega)$ is the FT of $E(t)$.[19] For simplicity and convenience, the term $\exp(j \cdot \omega_c \cdot t)$, where ω_c is the center frequency of the input laser, has been dropped. In the time domain, the reflected pulse envelope can then be expressed as $E_{Refl}(t) = E(t) * h_R(t)$, where '$*$' stands for the convolution operation. Therefore, the reflected pulse's complex electric field envelope is simply a convolution of the reflection impulse response of the FBG with the input pulse's complex electric field. If the pulsed laser field is temporally much narrower than the impulse response of the FBG, then the reflected pulse from the grating ideally becomes the impulse response itself, i.e., $h_R(t)$.

Returning to the first approach (Fig. 1(a)), the input laser pulse can be generated by a mode-locked laser and have a few ps temporal width. First, this input pulse is split into two arms, i.e., pulse A and B by use of a coupler, which has a splitting ratio of R, where R can range anywhere from for instance 1 to 200 or even higher. In the lower arm of Fig. 1(a), pulse B is then directed towards the FBG of interest, and the reflected pulse from the FBG is collected using a circulator. If the input pulse A is temporally narrow enough with respect to the impulse response of the FBG, the reflected pulse $E_{Refl}(t)$ is essentially identical to $h_R(t)$. For most of the commercially used FBGs operating around 1550 nm, the temporal width of the reflection impulse response is on the order of 50-100 ps or longer; thus, in practice, a laser pulse width of a few ps acts as a delta function and $E_{Refl}(t) = h_R(t)$. Next, the reflected impulse response of the FBG, $h_R(t)$, is collinearly combined in the time domain with pulse A of the upper arm, $E_A(t)$, with a delay of τ in between the two pulses (Fig. 1(a)). This pulse sequence, $E_{Seq}(t) = E_A(t) + h_R(t - \tau)$, is then sent to an OSA, which yields the optical power spectrum or the square of the FT magnitude of sequence's complex electric field envelope, i.e., $\left| E_{Seq}(\omega) \right|^2$, where $E_{Seq}(\omega)$ is the FT of $E_{Seq}(t)$. From *only* the measured FT magnitude square, i.e., $\left| E_{Seq}(\omega) \right|^2$, we propose using SIMBA to recover $h_R(t)$. The principle of the recovery relies on the fact that $E_{Seq}(t)$ can be made close to an MPF by increasing the peak amplitude of $E_A(t)$, which makes its FT phase recoverable from only its FT magnitude i.e., from $\left| E_{Seq}(\omega) \right|$. As discussed in Chapter 5, in principle, the recovery could be achieved by using analytical Hilbert transformation[14]; however, we prefer the iterative error reduction algorithm,[15-17] for both simplicity and better noise performance.

Let us now illustrate the recovery of $E_{Refl}(t) = h_R(t)$ from only the measured quantity, $\left| E_{Seq}(\omega) \right|^2$ or $\left| E_{Seq}(\omega) \right|$ with a numerical example. To this end, we choose a strongly chirped asymmetric FBG, which makes the recovery a harder task. The theoretical magnitude and phase of the reflection coefficient of the arbitrarily chosen chirped FBG, which were calculated using the transfer matrix formalism of Ref. 3, are shown in Fig. 3. The reflection band of this FBG is ~4 nm wide, between ~1548 nm and ~1552 nm. The magnitude of the theoretical reflection impulse response of this FBG is also shown in Fig. 4, which is numerically computed by taking an inverse FT of $r(\omega)$. The temporal width of the reflection impulse response is ~ 300 ps. This broad temporal width is primarily due to the strong chirp of the reflection coefficient. Finally, as expected, the reflection impulse response of the FBG is causal (Fig. 4).

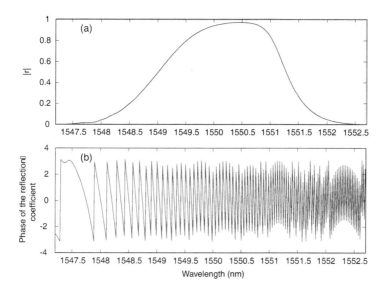

Fig. 3. The field reflection (a) magnitude and (b) phase of an asymmetric chirped FBG.

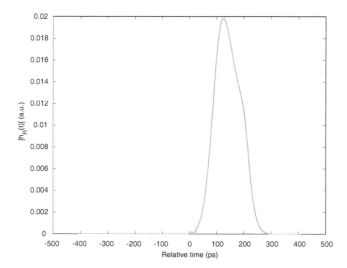

Fig. 4. Theoretical reflection impulse response of the chirped FBG shown in Fig. 3. Notice that due to the chirp of the FBG, the temporal width of its reflection impulse response is quite wide. Also note that, as expected, the reflection impulse response is causal.

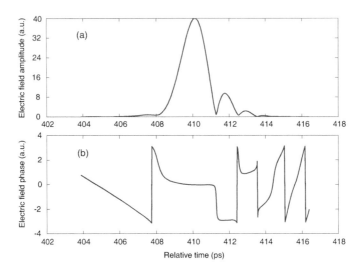

Fig. 5. Input laser pulse electric field envelope (a) magnitude, and (b) phase. Notice that the laser pulse actually acts as a delta function for the impulse response shown in Fig. 4.

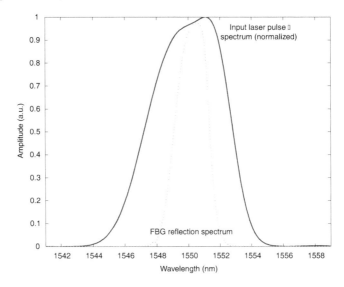

Fig. 6. Input laser pulse spectrum (normalized to one in amplitude) together with the reflection spectrum of the FBG shown in Fig. 3(a).

For the purpose of our numerical simulation, the temporal profile of the input laser pulse was chosen as shown in Fig. 5. The width of this pulse is less than ~ 6 ps, which essentially means that it acts as a delta function for the reflection impulse response of Fig. 4. The normalized magnitude of the input laser pulse spectrum, together with the reflection spectrum of the chosen FBG, are also plotted in Fig. 6. It should be noted that for the set-up of Fig. 1, the requirement for the input laser pulse is not only that its temporal width be much narrower than the impulse response of the FBG, i.e., it acts as a delta function, but also that its power spectrum covers all the frequencies in the FBG reflection spectrum. This is indeed the case in this numerical example as shown in Fig. 6.

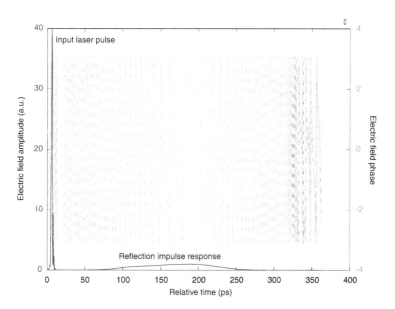

Fig. 7. Input pulse sequence formed using the set-up shown in Fig. 1. The solid curve is the electric field amplitude; the dashed curve is its phase. $\Re = 40$ is used for this numerical simulation to ensure that the complex electric field envelope of the pulse sequence is close to an MPF.

Using the set-up shown in Fig. 1(a), a sequence of two pulses is formed (Fig. 7). The first pulse, i.e., the input laser pulse, is followed by a weaker pulse reflected from the FBG, which essentially is the reflection impulse response of the FBG. The ratio of the peak amplitude of the input laser pulse to the peak amplitude of the reflection impulse response of the FBG, i.e., $\Re = \max(|E_A(t)|) / \max(|h_R(t)|)$, where 'max' defines the maximum value of the argument function, is crucial for our approach. In Fig. 7, $\Re = 40$ ensured that the complex electric field envelope of the pulse sequence is close to an MPF, which is a key requirement for SIMBA.

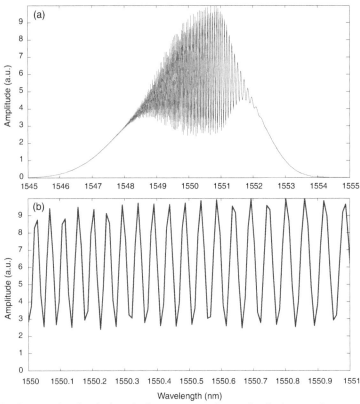

Fig. 8. (a) Output of a classical optical spectrum analyzer, for the input pulse sequence shown in Fig. 7. (b) Magnified view of a portion of the same plot as in (a). The resolution of the spectrum analyzer was assumed to be ~10 pm.

The pulse sequence of Fig. 7 is then sent to an OSA to record the power spectrum or the square of the FT magnitude of pulse sequence's complex electric field envelope. This power spectrum (Fig. 8) was calculated numerically from Fig. 7 assuming that the resolution of the OSA was only ~10 pm, which is actually a modest resolution for current state-of-the-art spectrum analyzers. The enlarged view of the same power spectrum between 1550 nm and 1551 nm (Fig. 8(b)) illustrates that due to the low resolution of the OSA, some sharp features are actually lost. As will be shown below, this limitation still enables us to recover the whole complex spectrum of the FBG accurately. The fringe pattern observed in Fig. 8 is the result of interference between the input laser pulse spectra and the FBG reflection spectra. This interference is only observed in the frequency band of the reflection spectrum of the FBG. The overall envelope of the power spectrum in Fig. 8(a) follows the power spectrum of the input laser pulse shown in Fig. 6.

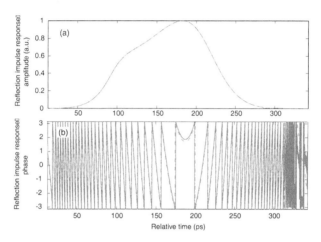

Fig. 9. (a) Normalized amplitude and (b) phase of the recovered reflection impulse response (the dashed line) of the FBG shown in Fig. 3. The solid curves are the amplitude and phase of the original theoretical impulse response. The recovery is close to being perfect.

The complex reflection impulse response of the target FBG can be recovered by feeding the iterative error-reduction algorithm described in Chapter 5 with the OSA output of Fig. 8(a). As can be seen in Fig. 9, the recovery is very good. At this point, we should mention that the time origin for the recovered impulse response is lost in Fig. 9. In principle, the time origin can be redefined by simply using the causality property of the impulse response, i.e., by choosing it as the point to the left of which the recovered impulse response is all zero. Any error in the redefinition of the time origin is, however, inconsequential, since a time shift in the impulse response adds a linear phase to its FT phase, and therefore, the recovered group delay $(d\phi/d\omega)$ will only have a *constant* offset, proportional to the error made in the recovery of the time origin. For practical applications, this constant group delay offset is inconsequential because it can simply be removed by subtracting the value of the group delay far away from the center wavelength of the FBG from the whole recovered group delay spectrum.

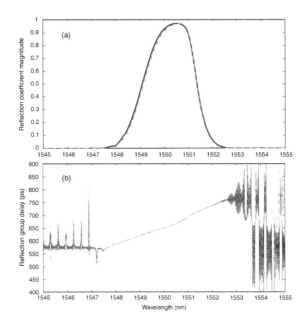

Fig. 10. Recovered (a) magnitude and (b) group delay spectra of the reflection coefficient of the FBG shown in Fig. 3. The recovered curves are shown with the dashed lines; the original curves are shown with the solid lines.

In Fig. 9, the recovery of the leading input pulse electric field is not shown, since it is not of interest. As also illustrated in Chapter 5, the input laser pulse simply acts as a dummy pulse for the recovery. In other words, the recovery of the reflection impulse response of the FBG is achieved at the cost of losing the leading input laser pulse's electric field information. However, because the input laser pulse profile is not our target, this is inconsequential .

From the recovered impulse response of the FBG (Fig. 9), the reflection coefficient magnitude and the group delay spectra of the same FBG can easily be computed by a single FT operation, the results of which are shown in Fig. 10. Even for a strongly chirped FBG (Fig. 3), the success in the recovery is quite impressive. The error in the recovery of $|r(\omega)|$, defined as $\dfrac{\int \left| |r(\omega)| - |\hat{r}(\omega)| \right|^2 d\omega}{\int |r(\omega)|^2 d\omega}$, where $|r(\omega)|$ and $|\hat{r}(\omega)|$ are the

original and the recovered quantities, respectively, is only ~0.08%.

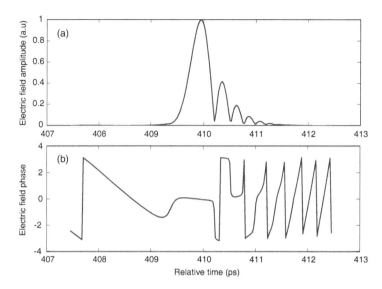

Fig. 11. Input laser pulse's normalized electric field envelope (a) magnitude and (b) phase. This pulse is temporally narrower by a factor of ~3 times than the laser pulse shown in Fig. 5.

To evaluate the dependence of the success of the recovery on the temporal profile of the chosen input laser pulse, we tested it with an input laser pulse (Fig. 11) ~3 times narrower than the input laser pulse used in the previous example (compare Figs. 5 and 11). In this numerical simulation $\Re = 120$ was used. The reason for the change in $\Re$ from 40 to 120 will be discussed in the discussion below. The FBG reflection coefficient magnitude and group delay spectra recovered in this case are shown in Fig. 12. The error in the recovery of $|r(\omega)|$ was reduced by more than a factor of 4, to less than 0.02%. This improved performance is primarily due to the narrower input laser pulse which acts more like a true delta function, yielding a more accurate reflected pulse that represents the true reflection impulse response of the FBG.

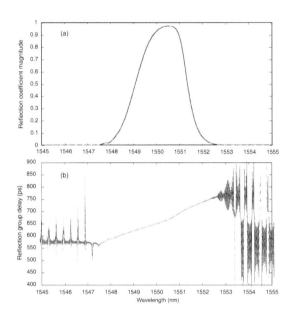

Fig. 12. Recovered (a) magnitude and (b) group delay spectra of the reflection coefficient of the FBG of Fig. 3, using the narrower laser pulse of Fig. 11 and $\Re$ = 120. The recovered curves are shown with the dashed lines; the original curves are shown with the solid lines. The recovery is improved to be excellent (compare with the recovery shown in Fig. 10).

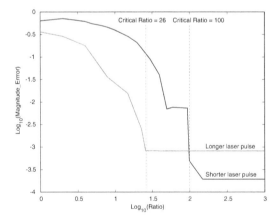

Fig. 13. Logarithmic error in the recovered magnitude of the reflection spectrum of the FBG, as a function of the logarithm of $\Re$.

To expand on the reason for the increase in $\Re$ (from 40 to 120), we ran a series of simulations for each of the two input laser pulses (longer and shorter pulses) shown in Figs. 5 and 11, respectively, and recorded the error in the recovery of $|r(\omega)|$ as a function of $\Re$. The results of this simulation are shown in Fig. 13. There are two important differences between the longer dummy pulse and the shorter dummy pulse simulations shown in Fig. 13. First, the shorter input pulse yields a much better recovery (the error is reduced by a factor of ~4) than the longer laser pulse, provided that a sufficiently large $\Re$ value is used. This observed lower baseline in error (Fig. 13) is simply due to the fact that, as briefly noted above, the shorter laser pulse acts more like a true delta function, yielding a more accurate representation of the true reflection impulse response of the FBG. This more accurate representation of $h_R(t)$ reduces the error in the recovery. It is interesting to note that the error is lowered by a factor of ~4 by using an input laser pulse that is temporally ~3 times narrower.

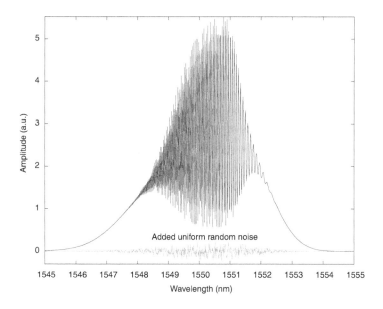

Fig. 14. Noisy output of the spectrum analyzer, where 10% peak-to-peak uniform random noise (also shown at the bottom) is added to the theoretical spectrum. The resolution of the spectrum analyzer was assumed to be ~10 pm and $\Re = 27$.

The second noteworthy difference in Fig. 13 is that the convergence of the error-reduction algorithm is achieved for a lower $\Re$ in the case of longer input pulse. Specifically, the critical $\Re$ for the longer pulse is only ~26, compared to ~100 for the shorter pulse (Fig. 13). In other words, using a narrower dummy input pulse requires a stronger peak amplitude (or a higher critical ratio) for the input pulse. An important parameter that will help the reader understand this behavior is simply the ratio of the integral of the normalized input laser field to the integral of the normalized reflection impulse response of the FBG, i.e., $\int \frac{|E_{Pulse}(t)|}{max(|E_{Pulse}(t)|)} dt / \int \frac{|h_R(t)|}{max(|h_R(t)|)} dt$. This ratio is 0.35% for the shorter pulse, and 1.4% for the longer pulse. In other words, for the shorter laser pulse, the total area under the normalized electric field magnitude is only 0.35% of the total area under the normalized magnitude of the reflection impulse response of the target FBG. This low ratio is expected, since the input laser pulse is required to act as a delta function. Interestingly, as this area ratio increases from 0.35% for the shorter pulse to 1.4% (i.e., by a factor of 4) for the longer pulse, the critical $\Re$ also drops by a factor of ~4, from 100 to 26. We conclude that for broader impulse response FBGs (such as strongly chirped FBGs), a larger critical $\Re$ is usually required to achieve convergence. This behavior is also related to an important property of MPFs, which states that most of the energy of an MPF is concentrated around *the origin*.[14] Therefore, the broader the reflection impulse response of the FBG, the more the peak amplitude of the leading dummy pulse must be increased to make this MPF property hold for the input pulse sequence.

Next, to address how measurement errors in the power spectrum affect the accuracy of FBG characterization, we multiplied the theoretical FT magnitude square of the input pulse sequence by a uniform random noise (*10% peak-to-peak amplitude with an average of unity*) to simulate a noisy spectrum (Fig. 14), and we applied SIMBA to it to recover the reflection impulse response of the target FBG. The reflection coefficient magnitude and the group delay spectra of the FBG were then computed by a simple FT operation. The result of this recovery is shown in Fig. 15. The recovery is still quite good in spite of the strong noise added. The large oscillations observed in the recovered group delay spectrum, especially towards the edges of the spectral window shown in Fig. 15(b), are simply due to the significant drop in the magnitude of the reflection coefficient at those wavelengths, which makes the recovery of spectral phase rather difficult. However this behavior is inconsequential, since the group delay in the most important wavelength range between 1548 nm and 1552 nm, is recovered quite well. In short, even with fairly noisy measurements, SIMBA works very well to characterize FBGs.

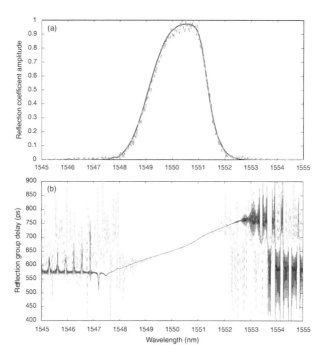

Fig. 15. Recovered (a) magnitude and (b) group delay spectra of the reflection coefficient of the FBG shown in Fig. 3, when a 10% peak-to-peak uniform random noise is added to the theoretical spectrum analyzer output, also shown in Fig. 14. The recovered curves are shown with the dashed lines; the original curves are shown with the solid lines.

As discussed in Chapter 5, the noise sensitivity of SIMBA is also affected by $\Re$. To maximize the accuracy of the recovery with noisy measurements, it is preferable to select an $\Re$ value close to the critical ratio; for this reason, we chose an $\Re$ value of 27 for the power spectrum shown in Fig. 14, which both ensured accurate convergence of the iterative error reduction algorithm and reduced sensitivity to measurement noise. In practice, the critical ratio that ensures the convergence can simply be traced by choosing two different $\Re$ values and comparing the difference between the recovery results, as also discussed in Chapter 5.

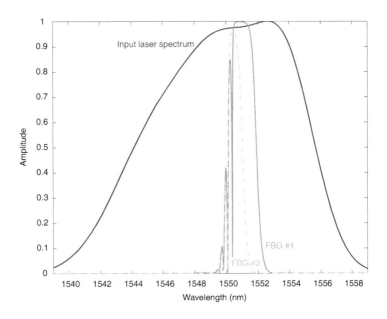

Fig. 16. Input laser pulse spectrum (normalized to one in amplitude) together with the reflection spectrum of two different FBGs.

So far, we have seen that for the proposed experimental set-up of Fig. 1, SIMBA can conveniently be used to uniquely characterize any FBG. This approach has important advantages with respect to existing techniques, e.g., low-coherence spectral interferometry. First, SIMBA gives two times better resolution than low-coherence spectral interferometry would yield using the same set-up. The reason is that in low-coherence spectral interferometry, by filtering in the inverse FT domain, the convolution of the impulse response with the auto-correlation function of the input laser pulse is recovered,[12,13] whereas using SIMBA, the convolution of the same impulse response with the input laser pulse itself is recovered. This constitutes an improved resolution of ~2 times. Second, the time delay between the input laser pulse and the reflection impulse response of the FBG can be made arbitrarily small, as long as there is no temporal overlap between the two pulses. Low-coherence spectral interferometry, in contrast, requires a certain minimum delay between these two pulses to ensure individual filtering of the above-mentioned convolution term in the IFT domain.[12,13] This becomes especially critical if the used OSA has low resolution. In that case, choosing a large time delay required by low-coherence spectral interferometry may result in rapid fringes in the power spectrum that the OSA cannot resolve. This can potentially cause severe recovery errors. The third significant advantage of our approach is that the recovery using SIMBA is more robust to noise and errors present in the measurement system. This improvement is simply because SIMBA works with $\left|E_{Seq}(\omega)\right|$, while all other spectral interferometry techniques work with $\left|E_{Seq}(\omega)\right|^2$, whose noise term is stronger.

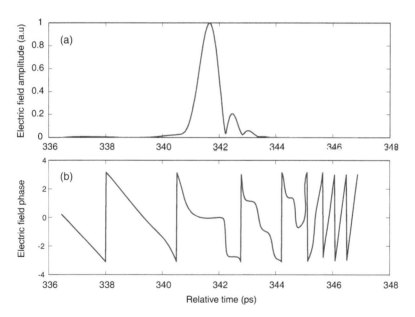

Fig. 17. Input laser pulse's normalized electric field envelope (a) magnitude and (b) phase. The amplitude spectrum of this pulse is also shown in Fig. 16.

A fourth important advantage of SIMBA over other techniques is that it can conveniently be used to simultaneously characterize multiple FBGs, using a single OSA measurement. For this purpose the same set-up shown in Fig. 1(a) can still be used, provided that the additional FBGs are added in a parallel fashion next to the first FBG. This way, the reflection impulse responses of all the FBGs can be time delayed with respect to the stronger dummy laser pulse. This pulse sequence, which now consists of more than 2 pulses, is again sent to an OSA for its power spectrum measurement. The measured power spectrum is processed as described above, i.e., using the iterative error reduction algorithm. To illustrate the success of the proposed multiple FBG characterization scheme in our numerical simulation, we have used the two Gaussian apodized FBGs shown in Fig. 16. The normalized magnitude spectrum and the temporal electric field profile of the input laser pulse are also shown in Fig. 16 and Fig. 17, respectively.

The pulse sequence, formed by time delaying the two reflected pulses from FBG#1 and FBG#2 with respect to the leading dummy input laser pulse, is also shown in Fig. 18. $\Re = 40$ was chosen for the simulation (Fig. 18). For this sequence of three pulses, the power spectrum is shown in Fig. 19. Once again, the resolution of the OSA was assumed to a modest number, i.e., ~10 pm. Using *only* the power spectrum measurement shown in Fig. 19, the reflection coefficient magnitude and group delay spectra for these two FBGs can be recovered simultaneously, as shown in Figs. 32 and 33, respectively. Once again, the recovery in both cases is very good, which proves that SIMBA can quite conveniently characterize multiple FBGs at once, using a single power spectrum measurement. The large-scale oscillations observed in the recovered group delay spectrum, especially towards the edges of the spectral window shown in for instance Fig. 20(b), are once again due to the significant drop in magnitude of the reflection coefficient at those wavelengths, which makes the recovery of spectral phase rather difficult. However, this difficulty is inconsequential, as discussed above relative to Fig. 15(b).

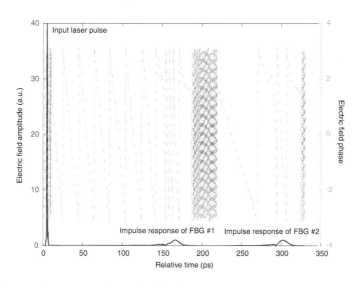

Fig. 18. Input pulse sequence formed using the set-up shown in Fig. 1. The solid line is the electric field magnitude; the dashed line is its phase. $\Re = 40$ for this numerical simulation. The reflected impulse response of the two FBGs follows the stronger input laser pulse.

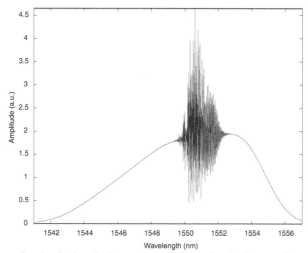

Fig. 19. Output of a classical optical spectrum analyzer, for the input pulse sequence shown in Fig. 18. The resolution of the spectrum analyzer was assumed to be ~10 pm. Also $\Re = 40$.

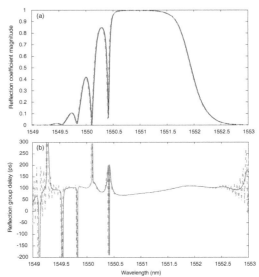

Fig. 20. Recovered (a) magnitude and (b) group delay spectra of the reflection coefficient of the FBG #1 shown in Fig. 16. The recovered curves are shown with the dashed lines; the original curves are shown with the solid lines.

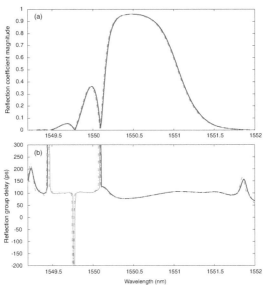

Fig. 21. Recovered (a) magnitude and (b) group delay spectra of the reflection coefficient of the FBG #2 shown in Fig. 16. The recovered curves are shown with the dashed lines; the original curves are shown with the solid lines.

7.3.2 THE SECOND PROPOSED SIMBA SET-UP FOR FBG CHARACTERIZATION

The second proposed set-up of SIMBA (Fig. 2), which shares all the benefits of the first approach discussed in the previous section, offers even more significant advantages over existing techniques. One of the most important additional features of the second approach is that the dummy input pulse does not need to be temporally much narrower than the reflection impulse response of the target FBG. As we have seen in the previous section, the first approach shown in Fig. 1, which gives a factor of two better resolution with respect to e.g., low-coherence spectral interferometry, uses an input dummy laser pulse that is ~50 times or more narrow than the reflection impulse response of the target FBG. In contrast, with this second approach, as will be demonstrated below, the same FBG can be characterized with an input laser pulse that is only ~2-5 times narrower than the reflection impulse response of the FBG.

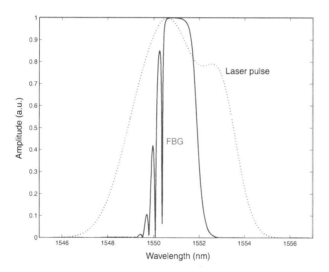

Fig. 22. Spectrum of the input laser pulse together with the reflection spectrum of the FBG of interest.

175

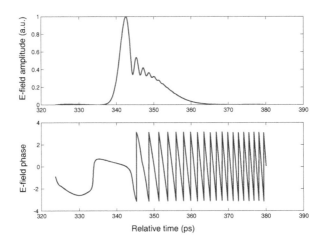

Fig. 23. Input laser pulse's normalized electric field envelope (a) magnitude and (b) phase. Normalized amplitude spectrum of this pulse is also shown in Fig. 22. The temporal width of this laser pulse is ~18 ps.

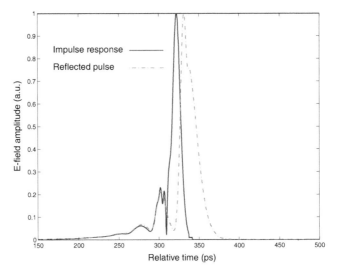

Fig. 24. A comparison between the magnitude of the impulse response of the FBG shown in Fig. 22, and the magnitude of the reflected pulse from the same FBG, when the time stretched pulse shown in Fig. 25 is incident to the FBG. The temporal width of the impulse response is ~37 ps, whereas the reflected pulse width is ~56 ps.

176

To illustrate how the second approach (Fig. 2) works with a numerical example, we will use the FBG reflection spectrum shown in Fig. 22. The latter figure also shows the normalized magnitude spectrum of the dummy input laser. The temporal profile of the input laser pulse (Fig. 23) reveals the width of the laser to be ~18 ps, where the temporal width is defined as the full width where the field reduces to 10% of its maximum value. The temporal width of the reflection impulse response of the same FBG is only wider by a factor of ~2, i.e., 37 ps (Fig. 24).

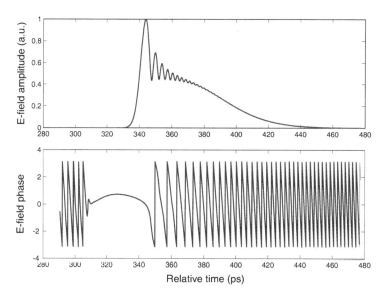

Fig. 25. Time-stretched laser pulse's normalized electric field envelope (a) magnitude and (b) phase. The temporal width of this stretched laser pulse is ~76 ps, which is ~4 times wider than the input laser pulse shown in Fig. 23.

As shown in Fig. 2, the input dummy laser pulse, 18 ps wide, is first split into two pulses, one of which is sent to a delay line, while the other is sent to a pulse stretcher that simply broadens the temporal width of the laser pulse by a factor of at least ~2-5. The pulse stretcher could, in principle, be a loop of single mode fiber optic cable that broadens the laser pulse width through dispersion. In our simulation, we assumed that the input laser pulse, which has a width of ~18 ps, is stretched in time by a factor of ~4, i.e., the time-stretched pulse width becomes ~76 ps (Fig. 25). It should be noted that the temporal electric field profile of the stretched pulse, i.e., $E_s(t)$, can be chosen arbitrarily, as long as it is wider than the dummy input laser pulse profile by a factor of *at least* 2-5 times.

Next, this broadened pulse is sent through an attenuator, and then split into two weak pulses as shown in Fig. 2. In our simulations, the attenuator was chosen to be ~32 dB (in power); however, it could be a value as low as ~20 dB. The reflected weak pulse from the target FBG is no longer the reflection impulse response of the FBG, since the incident pulse is much broader than the impulse response of the FBG. (Fig. 24) Actually, the reflected pulse is simply the convolution of the impulse response of the FBG with the temporal profile of the stretched pulse, i.e., $h_R(t) * E_s(t)$. The back reflections from the FBG and from the mirror (Fig. 2), which could, in principle, be a bare fiber end, are then temporally combined with the time-delayed version of the unattenuated initial dummy laser pulse in the lower arm of the set-up. This pulse sequence, which has a dominant peak pulse at the leading edge, followed by two weaker reflected pulses (Fig. 26), is then sent to an OSA to measure its power spectrum. Assuming a typical OSA with a resolution of ~10 pm, the theoretical power spectrum of the pulse sequence of Fig. 26 can be computed as shown in Fig. 27.

The processing of the measured output the OSA, as well as the principles of the recovery algorithm, are identical to the first approach discussed above. Because the input pulse sequence is close to an MPF, feeding the error reduction algorithm of Chapter 5 with *only* the OSA output (Fig. 27), both $E_s(t)$ and $h_R(t) * E_s(t)$ can be recovered simultaneously. Next, the reflection spectrum of the target FBG can simply be computed by taking the FTs of both $E_s(t)$ and $h_R(t) * E_s(t)$, i.e., $r(\omega) = \dfrac{FT\{h_R(t) * E_s(t)\}}{FT\{E_s(t)\}}$.

However, it is essential for the recovery that the power spectrum of the input laser pulse covers the frequency band of the target FBG (Fig. 22). Once again, the result of this recovery (Fig. 28) is very good. This result is quite exciting: using only *a single* OSA measurement, a Gaussian apodized FBG with an impulse response temporal width of ~37 ps has been fully characterized using a dummy laser pulse that has a temporal width of ~18 ps. The whole computation for the recovery process required only a few seconds to run, using MATLAB 5 on a 500 MHz computer.

Finally, as discussed in Chapter 5, various ultrashort pulse shaping techniques[20,21] can be used to modify the temporal profile of the dummy pulse to produce an absolutely true MPF for the pulse sequence's electric field to speed up the convergence of the results.

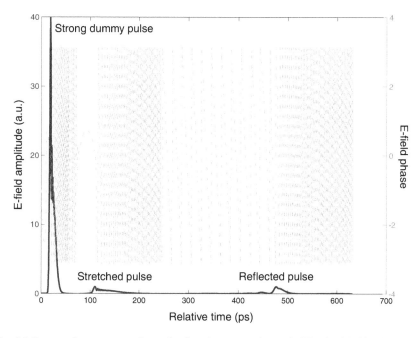

Fig. 26. Input pulse sequence formed using the set-up shown in Fig. 2 with $\Re = 40$. The reflected pulse from the FBG, together with the time-stretched laser pulse, follow the stronger input laser pulse.

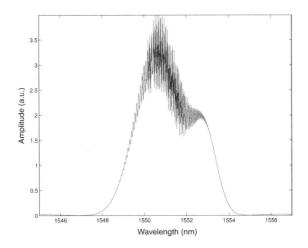

Fig. 27. Output of a classical optical spectrum analyzer for the input pulse sequence shown in Fig. 26. The resolution of the spectrum analyzer was assumed to be ~10 pm. A ratio of 40 was used between the peak amplitude of the input laser pulse and the peak amplitude of two pulses following the input pulse (Fig. 26).

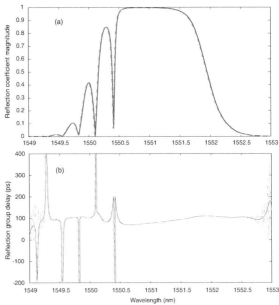

Fig. 28. Recovered (a) magnitude and (b) group delay spectra of the reflection coefficient of the FBG shown in Fig. 22. The recovered curves are shown with the dashed lines; the original curves are shown with the solid lines.

7.4 CONCLUSIONS

In this chapter, we discussed an interferometric approach that utilizes Spectral Interferometry using Minimum-phase Based Algorithms (SIMBA) to fully characterize magnitude and group delay spectra of *any* fiber Bragg grating, operating in transmission or reflection. This technique involves sending a laser pulse, e.g., a few ps temporal width, to the Bragg grating of interest and recording the spectrum of the interference between the reflected pulse from the grating and the time-delayed version of the original short pulse. This spectrum, which yields only the Fourier transform (FT) magnitude of the input pulse sequence's electric field envelope is then processed to uniquely recover both the phase and amplitude of the fiber Bragg grating spectrum. This is a quite important result since by only measuring an FT magnitude, the whole complex spectrum of the grating is recovered. Some important advantages of this approach with respect to the currently existing tools include (1) higher resolution, (2) better noise performance, (3) better compatibility with low-resolution OSA measurement systems, (4) the ability to characterize multiple FBGs all at once using a single measurement, and (5) the ability to work with longer duration input laser pulses.

REFERENCES

1. A. Othonos and K. Kalli, Fiber Bragg gratings: fundamentals and applications in telecommunications and sensing, (Artech House, Boston, 1999)

2. R. Kashyap, Fiber Bragg gratings, (Academic Press, San Diego, 1999)

3. T. Erdogan, "Fiber grating spectra," J. Lightwave Technol. 15, 1277 (1997)

4. L. Poladian, "Group-delay reconstruction for fiber Bragg gratings in reflection and transmission", Opt. Lett. 22, 1571 (1997)

5. A. Ozcan, M. J. F. Digonnet, and G. S. Kino, "Group delay recovery using iterative processing of amplitude of transmission spectra of fibre Bragg gratings," Electron. Lett. 40, 1104 (2004)

6. D. W. Huang and C. C. Yang, "Reconstruction of fiber grating refractive-index profiles from complex Bragg reflection spectra," Appl. Opt. 38, 4494 (1999)

7. J. Skaar, "Measuring the group delay of fiber Bragg gratings by use of end-reflection interference," Opt. Lett. 24, 1020 (1999)

8. P. Lambelet, P. Y. Fonjallaz, H. G. Limberger, R. P. Salathe, C. H. Zimmer, and H. H. Gilgen, "Bragg grating characterization by optical low-coherence reflectometry," IEEE Photon. Technol. Lett. 5, 565 (1993)

9. U. Wiedmann, P. Gallion, G. Duan, "A Generalized approach to optical low-coherence reflectometry inducing spectral filtering effects," J. of Lightwave Technol. 16, 1343 (1998)

10. E. I. Petermann, J. Skaar, B. E. Sahlgreen, R. A. H. Stubbe, A. T. Friberg, "Characterization of fiber Bragg gratings by use of optical coherence-domain reflectometry," J. of Lightwave Technol. 17, 2371 (1999)

11. S. D. Dyer, K. B. Rochford and A. H. Rose, "Fast and accurate low-coherence interferometric measurements of fiber Bragg grating dispersion and reflectance," Optics Express 5, 262 (1999)

12. S. Keren and M. Horowitz, "Interrogation of fiber gratings by use of low-coherence spectral interferometry of noiselike pulses," Opt. Lett. 26, 328 (2001)

13. S. Keren, A. Rosenthal, and M. Horowitz, "Measuring the structure of highly reflecting fiber Bragg gratings," IEEE Photon. Tech. Lett. **15**, 575 (2003)

14. V. Oppenheim and R. W. Schafer, *Digital Signal Processing*, (Prentice Hall, 2002), Chap. 7.

15. T. F. JR. Quatieri and A. V. Oppenheim, "Iterative techniques for minimum phase signal reconstruction from phase or magnitude," IEEE Transactions on Acoustics, Speech, and Signal Processing 29, 1187 (1981)

16. M. Hayes, J. S. Lim, and A. V. Oppenheim, "Signal reconstruction from phase or magnitude," IEEE Trans. Acoust., Speech, Signal Processing **28**, 672 (1980).

17. A. Ozcan, M. J. F. Digonnet, and G. S. Kino, "Iterative processing of second-order optical nonlinearity depth profiles," Opt. Express 12, 3367 (2004), http://www.opticsexpress.org/abstract.cfm?URI=OPEX-12-15-3367

18. J. Skaar, "Synthesis of fiber Bragg gratings for use in transmission," J. Opt. Soc. Am. A **18**, 557 (2001)

19. L. R. Chen, S. D. Benjamin, P. W. E. Smith and J. E. Sipe, "Ultrashort pulse reflection from fiber gratings: a numerical investigation," J. of Lightwave Technol. **15**, 1503 (1997)

20. M. M. Wefers and K. A. Nelson, "Analysis of programmable ultrashort waveform generation using liquid-crystal spatial light modulators", J. Opt. Soc. Am. B **12**, 1343 (1995)

21. A. Rundquist, A.Efimov, and D. H. Reitze, "Pulse shaping with the Gerchberg-Saxton algorithm", J. Opt. Soc. Am. B **19**, 2468 (2002)

CHAPTER 8: APPLICATIONS OF MINIMUM PHASE FUNCTIONS TO OPTICAL COHERENCE TOMOGRAPHY

In this chapter, we present a simple processing technique that uses, for the first time, the concept of minimum phase functions (MPFs) to improve frequency-domain optical coherence tomography (OCT) systems. This approach improves both the signal-to-noise ratio and measurement range, and requires a lower resolution optical spectrum analyzer than existing processing techniques.

8.1 INTRODUCTION

Optical coherence tomography, which is used in medicine to image tissues of various parts of the body,[1-10] consists of two major techniques: (1) time-domain OCT and (2) frequency-domain OCT. In both, a broadband light source, such as a superluminescent diode feeds an interferometer, typically a Michelson interferometer. The light signal is split into two fields using a beam splitter or a fiber coupler, as shown in Fig. 1; each field is directed towards one arm of the interferometer. In the lower arm (Fig. 1) a reference broadband mirror is placed, whereas in the other arm, the tissue of interest is placed. The reflected light from the tissue and the reference mirror are combined collinearly at the detector. In time-domain OCT, the reference mirror is moveable, and is scanned during the image acquisition. In frequency-domain OCT, the reference mirror is fixed. At the detector end of frequency-domain OCT, the spectrum of the interference between the two reflected signals (coming from each arm of the interferometer) is recorded by an optical spectrum analyzer (OSA). As will be further explored in the next section, because the reference mirror acts as a true delta function (spatially), this recorded power spectrum yields the complex scattering function of the tissue of interest under certain set of conditions. Frequency-domain OCT demonstrates significant advantages over time-domain OCT, including higher speed and better sensitivity.[1,7,8]

In this chapter, we apply the concepts of MPFs to improve frequency-domain OCT systems. The proposed improvements are based on our discovery that the effective complex tissue scattering function in the conventional OCT systems is an MPF. Based on this, we propose a simple processing technique for the conventional frequency-domain OCT set-up that enables a better signal-to-noise ratio, an improved measurement range, and that requires a lower resolution optical spectrum analyzer than existing processing techniques.[4-10] This also reduces both the cost of the OCT system and the image acquisition time for the same signal-to-noise ratio. As in previous chapters, our approach relies on the property of minimum phase functions, which make it possible to recover a function, complex in this case, from *only* its Fourier transform (FT) magnitude.[11-17] As will be proved below, in a typical OCT set-up such as shown in Fig. 1, the effective complex scattering function, which by definition is a linear summation of the tissue and the reference mirror scattering functions, is an MPF or close to being one, and this property allows us to recover it by means of either the analytical Hilbert transformation or the iterative processing of the measured power spectrum data.[11-17] Both the analytical Hilbert transform and the iterative processing approaches are limited to minimum phase functions.

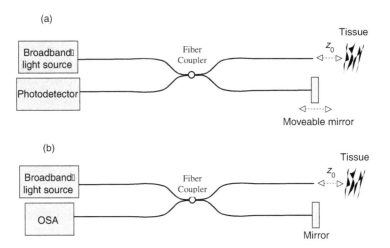

Fig. 1. Generic block diagram of (a) time-domain OCT; (b) frequency-domain OCT.

8.2 FREQUENCY-DOMAIN OCT USING MINIMUM PHASE FUNCTIONS

Before discussing the improvements that the use of MPF concepts brings to OCT, we first analyze the classical frequency-domain OCT set-up in greater detail. For Fig. 1(b), let us assume that the complex field scattering function (sometimes also called the scattering potential,[1]) of the tissue of interest is $f(z)$, where z is the depth into the tissue, confined to the $z \geq 0$ half space. Let us also assume that the spectral intensity distribution of the broadband source is given by $S(k)$, where $k = 2\pi/\lambda$ and λ is the wavelength of light. The detected signal at the OSA (Fig. 1(b)) is due to the interference of different frequency components reflecting from both the reference mirror and the tissue of interest. Mathematically, this recorded power spectrum can be written as:

$$I(k') = S(k') \cdot \left| \int_{-\infty}^{\infty} g(z) \cdot \exp(jk' 2n_T z) \cdot dz \right|^2 \quad (1)$$

where $g(z) = R \cdot \delta(z) + f(z - z_0)$, $\delta(z)$ is the spatial Dirac-delta function, $k' = k - 2\pi/\lambda_0$, λ_0 is the center frequency of $S(k)$, R is the field reflectivity of the reference mirror, z_0 is the offset distance between the reference arm and the tissue arm, as shown in Fig. 1(b), and n_T is the refractive index of the tissue, where the dispersion of the tissue has been ignored, i.e., $n_T(k) \approx n_T$. This last assumption is quite safe, and has also been used in other treatments of OCT.[1,5] By defining the spatial FT frequency as $f = -k' \cdot n_T/\pi$, the expression in Eq. (1) then takes the form of an FT, i.e.,

$$I(f) = S(f) \cdot |G(f)|^2 \quad (2)$$

where $G(f)$ is the FT of $g(z)$. If the spectral bandwidth of the broadband source of Fig. 1 is sufficiently broad and smooth (which affects the resolution of the OCT system), then one can assume $S(f)$ to be constant across the spectrum of $G(f)$ such that $I(f) \approx s \cdot |G(f)|^2$, where s is a proportionality constant.

The classical frequency-domain OCT is based on a processing algorithm[4-10] that directly takes the inverse FT of Eq. (2). To present a *simple and fair* comparison of

187

our approach with conventional processing techniques,[4-10] we will assume that $S(f)$ is broad enough, i.e., $I(f) \approx |G(f)|^2$, where without loss of generality the constant s has been dropped. This assumption, which is frequently used in classical OCT analysis,[1] will not affect our conclusions, as it is also applied to the conventional processing techniques.

In the classical, well-established approach,[4-10] taking the IFT of the measured OSA spectrum, i.e., $I(f) \approx |G(f)|^2$, directly yields:

$$IFT\left\{|G(f)|^2\right\} = |R|^2 \cdot \delta(z) + A.C.\{f(z)\} + R \cdot f^*(-z-z_0) + R^* \cdot f(z-z_0) \quad (3)$$

where '$A.C.$' stands for the complex auto-correlation function and '$*$' for the complex conjugate operation. The important term for the recovery of the tissue scattering function is the last term, $R^* \cdot f(z-z_0)$. However, the $A.C.\{f(z)\}$ term in Eq. (3), which is centered around $z = 0$, usually obscures $R^* \cdot f(z-z_0)$ by spatial aliasing and it degrades the sensitivity and signal-to-noise ratio of the frequency-domain OCT systems[1,9]. In the classical processing approach, by choosing a large enough z_0, $R^* \cdot f(z-z_0)$ is shifted in space away from the origin, which reduces spatial aliasing with the $A.C.\{f(z)\}$ term. The complex scattering potential of the tissue of interest $f(z)$, is then recovered by filtering the $R^* \cdot f(z-z_0)$ term around $z = z_0$. For a broadband source with a coherence length of ~40 μm, a z_0 greater than 200 μm is sufficient to nearly eliminate the spatial overlap. However, choosing a sufficiently large z_0 leads to other problems. For instance, a large z_0 causes the fringes observed in the OSA spectrum to get closer, and a high-resolution OSA is required to resolve them. A large z_0 also reduces the maximum depth that can be probed in the tissue (for a given OSA). [1,9]

To improve the resolution, signal-to-noise ratio, and measurement range of the recovered images in frequency-domain OCT systems, we propose a simple processing approach that is based on MPFs.[11-17] The first relevant discovery is that the effective scattering function in an OCT system, i.e., $g(z) = R \cdot \delta(z) + f(z-z_0)$, has a dominant peak right at the origin, since for a typical tissue, where $n_T \approx 1.5$, $max\{|f(z)|\} << 1$, whereas $R \approx 1$. This directly implies that $g(z) = R \cdot \delta(z) + f(z - z_0)$ is either close to an MPF or an exact MPF, a property that makes it possible to recover $f(z)$, *uniquely*, from *only* the knowledge of $|G(f)|$, *regardless* of the value of z_0. As already discussed in Chapters 5 and 7, this recovery can be accomplished by either analytical or iterative approaches. For its better performance the iterative error-reduction algorithm, such as the Fienup[14] or the Gerchberg-Saxton[15] algorithm is again preferred. Given a complex MPF, $g(z)$, the only quantity that is fed into the iterative algorithm is the FT magnitude spectrum of $g(z)$. Similar to previous chapters, the initial guess for the missing FT phase can conveniently be chosen to be zero all across the spectrum.

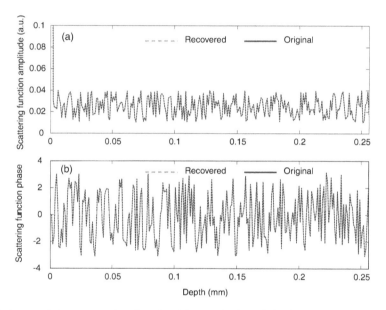

Fig. 2 Assumed tissue scattering function (a) magnitude and (b) phase (solid curves). For this simulation z_0 is assumed to be zero. The recovered scattering function is shown as the dashed curves. The recovery is so good that the two curves are indistinguishable.

Recovering $f(z)$ from *only* the knowledge of $|G(f)|$ using the above-mentioned MPF-based iterative algorithm has significant advantages over the conventional processing approaches[4-10]. First, there is no minimum constraint on z_0, which means that z_0 can conveniently be chosen close to 0. This change implies that for the same performance a lower resolution OSA can now be used, which also reduces both the cost of the OCT system and the image acquisition time for the same signal-to-noise ratio level. Furthermore, since the depth measurement range into the tissue is inversely proportional to the maximum spatial frequency measured in the OSA spectrum,[1] in principle, a z_0 close to 0 allows a greater measurement range for the OCT set-up. Second, while conventional approaches take a direct IFT of $I(k')$, our technique uses the square root of the measured power spectrum, i.e., $\sqrt{I(k')}$. Since the noise term in $I(k')$ is stronger than in $\sqrt{I(k')}$, our technique outperforms the conventional approach for noise sensitivity. Finally, the degradation in the signal-to-noise ratio associated with spatial aliasing due to the $A.C.\{f(z)\}$ term completely disappears in our MPF-based processing.

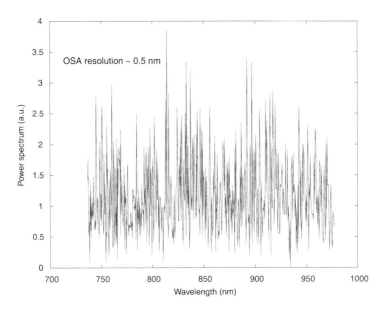

Fig. 3 Theoretical power spectrum of the OCT set-up, computed for the scattering function of Fig. 2. The resolution of the OSA in the OCT set-up was assumed to be limited by ~0.5 nm.

Now, let us show the strength of our approach using numerical simulations. For the first numerical simulation, we assumed $z_0 = 0$, which means that the length of the upper arm is roughly matched to the length of the lower arm of the Michelson interferometer in the OCT set-up (Fig. 1). To simulate a more challenging problem, we assumed that the complex tissue scattering function is a uniform random variable (both in magnitude and phase), as shown in Figs. 2(a) and 2(b), respectively. For this simulation, the finite size of the laser spot at the tissue has been ignored such that the reflected beams are assumed to be plane waves. However, this assumption has no effect on the axial resolution along z. The field reflectivity of the tissue varies in magnitude between 0.01 and 0.04. These numbers are not critical for our technique and could be chosen differently. The mirror reflectivity is $R = 1$. The sharp peak near the origin (not fully shown in Fig. 2(a)) therefore climbs up to 1. Note also that the whole cross section of the tissue is assumed to be ~0.25 mm. Once again, this number could as well be chosen larger or smaller without any change in the results.

To simulate the output of the OSA, we computed numerically the power spectrum (the square of the FT magnitude) of the effective scattering function shown in Fig. 2. This spectrum is shown in Fig. 3. For this computation, a center wavelength of 840 nm is assumed for the broadband source. The entire trace shown in Fig. 3 has only 512 data points, which corresponds to a resolution of ~0.5 nm for the OSA. Feeding the square root of this power spectrum into the error reduction algorithm yields the recovered complex tissue scattering function shown in Fig. 2. The recovery for both the amplitude and the phase of the tissue scattering function is so good that the recovered curves cannot be distinguished from the original curves (Fig. 2). Using MATLAB 5 on a 500 MHz computer, the complete recovery took less than one second, which suggests that a faster programming environment such as C++, together with a faster processor, could yield ~ms computation times, and thus real time. A more careful choice of the initial FT phase could further speed up the convergence of the iterative algorithm, from, for instance, ~100 iterations to less than 10 iterations. For all the simulations shown in this chapter, a uniform zero FT phase has been assumed as the initial condition. However, in real tissue imaging, the FT phase determined by a first depth measurement can be used as the initial FT phase for the second depth measurement at a nearby spot along the tissue. Alternatively, the analytical Hilbert transformation of the square root of the power spectrum could be used to compute the initial FT phase. Even though this second approach is computationally challenging and more sensitive to noise, it can yield a better initial guess for the missing FT phase. Each of these methods has the potential to reduce the number of iterations required for convergence in a practical application to fewer than ~10.

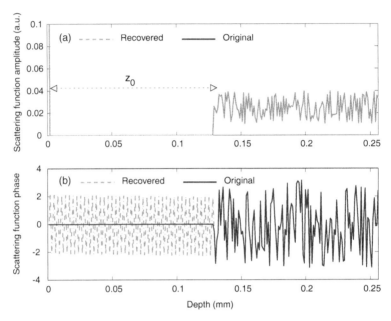

Fig. 4. Assumed tissue scattering function (a) magnitude and (b) phase (solid curves). For this simulation, z_0 is assumed to be ~0.12 mm. The recovered scattering function is shown with the dashed curves. The recovery in the tissue region (between ~0.12-0.25 mm) is so good that the two curves are indistinguishable. Notice that the recovered phase for the gap region (between ~0-0.12 mm) is not recovered, which is due to the fact that the magnitude of the function is identical to zero in this region. The concept of a definite phase is then meaningless anyway.

Next, we test our algorithm for a $z_0 \approx 1.2$ mm (Fig. 4), while maintaining the other parameters of the previous run (Fig. 2). The power spectrum of the complex tissue scattering function shown in Fig. 4 was computed numerically and is shown in Fig. 5. Since z_0 is now sizeable, the fringes in the power spectrum now oscillates more rapidly (compare Figs. 3 and 5). Once again, feeding the square root of this power spectrum to the iterative error reduction algorithm yields the recovered complex tissue scattering function shown in Fig. 4. The recovery is again excellent. The recovered phase of the tissue scattering function can simply be ignored in the gap region, i.e., between 0-0.12

mm, since the magnitude of the function in that interval is zero, making the definition of a definite phase meaningless.

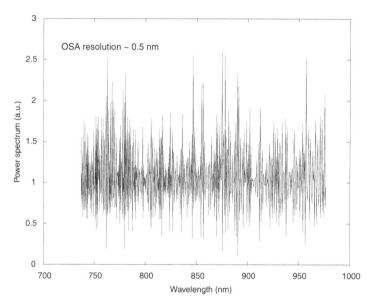

Fig. 5. Theoretical power spectrum of the OCT set-up, computed for the scattering function of Fig. 4. The resolution of the OSA in the OCT set-up was assumed to be limited to ~0.5 nm. Notice the higher frequency oscillations in the power spectrum compared with Fig. 3; which are due to the larger value of z_0 (~0.12 mm).

As discussed in Chapters 5 and 7, the ratio of R to $max\{|f(z)|\}$ is the critical parameter for the success of the recovery of our technique. This parameter determines how close the effective complex scattering function, $g(z) = R \cdot \delta(z) + f(z - z_0)$ is to a true MPF. In the simulations presented so far, this ratio was $1 / 0.04 = 25$. Since the scattering function is quite weak for typical tissue samples, a ratio of 25 is a reasonable assumption. However, for cases where $max\{|f(z)|\} \ll 1$ cannot be satisfied, this ratio can easily be increased by using an uneven beam splitter or an attenuator in the OCT set-up. We have found empirically that a ratio of greater than ~10 will always converge. To briefly show what happens to the recovery when R is reduced to 0.2 while still keeping $max\{|f(z)|\} = 0.04$, i.e., a ratio of 5, the results of the recovery of the complex tissue scattering function is plotted in Fig. 6. As one can see, the recovery in this case is not acceptable due to the lower value of the $R/max\{|f(z)|\}$ ratio.

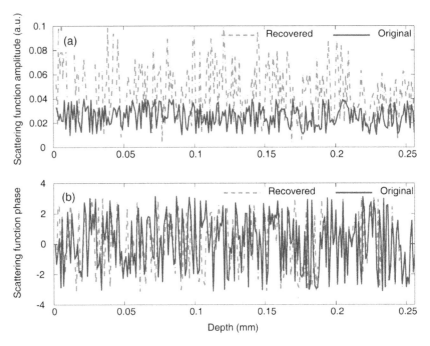

Fig. 6. Assumed tissue scattering function (a) magnitude and (b) phase (solid curves). For this simulation z_0 is assumed to be zero, and $R = 0.2$. The recovered scattering function is shown with the dashed curves. The recovery is not acceptable in this case due to the low value (5) of the $R/max\{|f(z)|\}$ ratio.

We now briefly comment on the reference mirror used in the lower arm of the Michelson interferometer shown in Fig. 1(b). Ideally, the spatial scattering (reflection) function of the assumed broadband mirror is a Dirac-delta function. However, for our approach it does not have to be a true delta function, e.g., a stacked dielectric mirror or even a fiber Bragg grating with a broader spatial scattering function could also be used. In that case the effective tissue scattering function can be written as $g(z) = R(z) + f(z - z_0)$, where $R(z)$ is the reflectivity of the reference arm as a function of space. We have found empirically that the MPF-based iterative algorithm still converges to the unique solution as long as $R(z)$ is much narrower than the width of $f(z)$, for instance by a factor of ~5 or more. To illustrate, for a tissue thickness of 0.5 mm, a reference mirror with a spatial scattering function width of ~100 μm or less could safely be used. For typical metal-coated reference mirrors, the spatial width will, in effect, be less than 1 micron, acting almost like a true Dirac-delta function, ($R(z) = R \cdot \delta(z)$) which is the ideal situation for our processing approach.

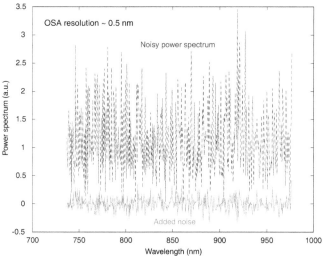

Fig. 7. The power spectrum of a noisy OCT set-up. The added noise (also shown at the bottom) is a 30% peak-to-peak amplitude uniform random noise. The resolution of the OSA in the OCT set-up was assumed to be ~0.5 nm.

Next, we added a *30%* peak-to-peak amplitude uniform random noise to the theoretical power spectrum (Fig. 7) to show how measurement errors and noise in the power spectrum affect the accuracy of the profiles recovered with our technique. The resolution of the OSA was again limited to ~0.5 nm; all other parameters were the same as in the simulation of Fig. 2. In this noisy case, the recovered complex scattering function of the tissue is shown in Fig. 8. The recovery results for both the phase and amplitude of the complex scattering function is quite impressive: even under 30% uniform random noise, almost all the details of the scattering potential have still been recovered faithfully, which demonstrates that our approach can be used confidently, even in a fairly noisy OCT set-up.

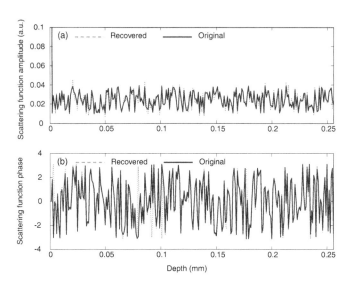

Fig. 8. Assumed tissue scattering function (a) magnitude and (b) phase (solid curves). For this simulation a *30%* peak-to-peak amplitude uniform random noise is added to the theoretical power spectrum (Fig. 7). The recovered scattering function is shown with the dashed curves. Even with considerable noise, the recovery accuracy is still quite respectable.

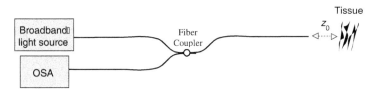

Fig. 9. An alternative frequency-domain OCT set-up that does not involve a separate arm for the interferometer.

At this point, we discuss the possibility of using a simpler set-up than the classical frequency-domain OCT set-up shown in Fig. 1(b). Our MPF-based approach requires a large but easy-to-realize $R/max\{|f(z)|\}$ ratio (e.g., >10), which could be achieved with a simpler set-up as shown in Fig. 9. For *weakly reflecting tissues*, instead of a reference mirror in a separate arm, we propose to use the fiber end as the reference mirror. In this new configuration (Fig. 9), the effective complex scattering function will *still* be in the form $g(z) = R \cdot \delta(z) + f(z - z_0)$. However, since for a bare fiber end in air, $R \sim 0.2$, this set-up will be limited to weakly reflecting tissues such that $max\{|f(z)|\} \lesssim \sim 0.02$. If this condition is satisfied, then $g(z) = R \cdot \delta(z) + f(z - z_0)$ will be close enough to a true MPF that our technique can safely be applied to uniquely image the complex scattering function of the tissue. In the worst case, $max\{|f(z)|\} \leq \sim 0.02$ condition can be realized by placing either a broadband attenuator (that can be tilted to avoid multiple reflections) just in front of the tissue, or a coated fiber end to increase the value of R. However, for applications where a contact between the fiber end and the tissue is desired these two approaches will fail.

Finally, using an angled fiber end in Fig. 9, ($R = 0$) would mean that there is no interference at the OSA. In that case, the measured quantity will be the power spectrum of the tissue's complex scattering function, $f(z)$, i.e., $|F(f)|^2$. However, due to the high reflection from the air-tissue interface, $f(z)$ will, *in most cases*, have a sharp peak close to the origin. This would make $f(z)$ close to an MPF, i.e., the whole complex $f(z)$ can be fully recovered from only the measurement of $|F(f)|^2$, using the analytical Hilbert transformation or the iterative error reduction algorithm discussed above. The only exception to this simple approach would be special tissues, where there is a strong scattering source in the deeper part of the tissue. In that case, $f(z)$ may not be an MPF, and hence an interferometric set-up ($R > 0$) is needed. However, we believe that the above-mentioned simple approach based on MPFs is still an important opportunity for fast imaging of a wide range of tissues.

8.3 CONCLUSIONS

This chapter describes a powerful processing technique based on minimum phase functions, to improve frequency-domain OCT systems. Rather than taking a direct IFT of the recorded power spectrum (as in the classical OCT technique), our solution uses iterative processing of the square root of the power spectra to uniquely recover the complex effective scattering function of the tissue. Using numerical simulations, we have shown that this iterative approach works very well, even with fairly high noise levels. Our approach improves both the signal-to-noise ratio and measurement range, and requires a lower resolution optical spectrum analyzer than existing processing techniques. As a result of this, both the cost of the OCT system and the image acquisition time for the same signal-to-noise ratio level are also reduced. To our knowledge, this is the first time that minimum-phase functions have been used to improve optical coherence tomography systems.

REFERENCES

1. T. Asakura, *International trends in optics and photonics ICO IV*, (Springer-Verlag, Berlin Heidelberg, 1999), pp. 359-389

2. D. Huang, *et al.* "Optical coherence tomography," Science 254, 1178 (1991)

3. J. G. Fujimoto, *et al.* "Optical biopsy and imaging using optical coherence tomography," Nature Medicine 1, 970 (1995)

4. A. F. Fercher, C. K. Hitzenberger, G. Kamp, and S. Y. El-Zaiat, "Measurement of intraocular distances by backscattering spectral interferometry," Opt. Commun. 117, 43 (1995)

5. G. Hausler and M. W. Lindler, "Coherence radar and spectral radar- New tools for dermatological diagnosis," J. Biomed. Opt. 3, 21 (1998)

6. M. Wojtkowski, R. A. Leitgeb, A. Kowalczyk, T. Bajraszewski, and A. F. Fercher, "In vivo human retinal imaging by Fourier domain optical coherence tomography", J. Biomed. Opt. 7, 457, (2003)

7. R. A. Leitgeb, C. K. Hitzenberger, and A. F. Fercher, "Performance of Fourier domain vs. time-domain optical coherence tomography", Optics Express 11, 889, (2003)

8. M. A. Choma, M. V. Sarunic, C. Yang, and J. A. Izatt, "Sensitivity advantage of swept source and Fourier domain optical coherence tomography," Optics Express 11, 2183, (2003)

9. R. A. Leitgeb, C. K. Hitzenberger, A. F. Fercher, and T. Bajraszewski "Phase-shifting algorithm to achieve high-speed long-depth-range probing by frequency-domain optical coherence tomography," Opt. Lett. 28, 2201, (2003)

10. R. A. Leitgeb, *et al.* "Ultrahigh resolution Fourier domain optical coherence tomography", Optics Express 12, 2156, (2004)

11. V. Oppenheim and R. W. Schafer, *Digital Signal Processing*, (Prentice Hall, 2002), Chap. 7.

12. T. F. Quatieri, Jr., and A. V. Oppenheim, "Iterative techniques for minimum phase signal reconstruction from phase or magnitude," IEEE Trans. Acoust., Speech, Signal Processing 29, 1187 (1981)

13. M. Hayes, J. S. Lim, and A. V. Oppenheim, "Signal reconstruction from phase or magnitude," IEEE Trans. Acoust., Speech, Signal Processing 28, 672 (1980)

14. J. R. Fienup, "Reconstruction of an object from the modulus of its Fourier transform," Opt. Lett. 3, 27 (1978)

15. R. W. Gerchberg and W. O. Saxton, "Practical algorithm for the determination of phase from image and diffraction plane pictures," Optik 35, 237 (1972)

16. A. Ozcan, M. J. F. Digonnet, and G. S. Kino, "Iterative processing of second-order optical nonlinearity depth profiles," Opt. Express 12, 3367 (2004), http://www.opticsexpress.org/abstract.cfm?URI=OPEX-12-15-3367

17. A. Ozcan, M. J. F. Digonnet, and G. S. Kino, "Group delay recovery using iterative processing of amplitude of transmission spectra of fibre Bragg gratings," Electron. Lett. 40, 1104 (2004)

CHAPTER 9: OTHER POTENTIAL APPLICATIONS OF MINIMUM PHASE
FUNCTION CONCEPTS

This chapter explores other potential applications of minimum phase function (MPF) concepts, specifically, possible improvements in optical image processing, femtosecond spectroscopy and characterization of nonlinear coefficient profile of quasi-phase-matched (QPM) gratings are discussed. However, since the analysis required is similar to the treatment given in the earlier chapters, detailed proofs of concepts will not be presented in this chapter. For QPM grating characterization, Prof. Fejer of Applied Physics Department of Stanford University is acknowledged for his initial suggestion and useful discussions.

9.1 OPTICAL IMAGE PROCESSING

Minimum phase function concepts can also be applied to the broad field of optical image processing. We focus in particular on simple optical measurement systems that yield the Fourier transform (FT) of a two-dimensional complex object function, which can physically be any transparent object such as a photographic transparency, a spatial light modulator, or even a biological sample that modifies both the amplitude and the phase of the transmitted (or reflected) optical waves. One example of such an optical system is free-space propagation, i.e., the very well known far-field diffraction pattern (the Fraunhofer pattern), which yields the FT of the *complex* transmission function of an aperture that is illuminated with plane waves.[1] A thin converging lens is another example that yields the FT of a two-dimensional complex object function. At the focal plane of the lens, the formed image is the FT of the object function placed anywhere before the image plane, preferably at the front focal plane.[1] However, for both of the above-mentioned systems, the detected quantities are often only the FT magnitudes and the direct measurement of the phase is a difficult task.

MPF concepts can be used to uniquely recover the two-dimensional complex transmission function of the object of interest, $t_O(x, y)$, where x and y are the coordinates along the surface of the object, from *only* the image of its two-dimensional *FT magnitude.* For this purpose, we propose using a synthetic aperture, as shown in Fig. 1(a), with a complex transmission function of $t_A(x,y)$, placed next to the object of interest. The effective transmission function of the system can now be expressed as $t(x,y) = t_O(x,y) \cdot t_A(x,y)$. The synthetic aperture $t_A(x,y)$ was specially chosen to make the effective transmission function of the system close to an MPF for *any* choice of $t_O(x,y)$. To meet this goal, $t_A(x,y)$ has a small hole, which has transmission coefficient of unity, close to one of its corners with a diameter of D (Fig. 1(a)). The rest of the aperture can be partially transparent, with a uniform field transmission coefficient of ~30% or even less. To avoid multiple reflections between the object and aperture planes so that $t(x,y) = t_O(x,y) \cdot t_A(x,y)$ is valid, the synthetic aperture can be tilted slightly.

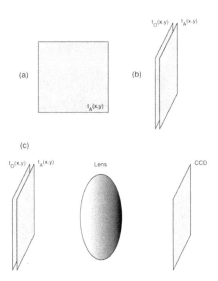

Fig. 1. (a) Cross section of the proposed synthetic aperture, where there is a small hole at one of its corners with 100% transmission, and the rest of the aperture is partially transparent. (b) The structure formed by pressing the synthetic aperture to the object of interest. The effective complex transmission function of this structure becomes close to an MPF, if not an exact MPF. (c) A typical imaging system that records the square of the FT magnitude of the object image.

The effect of the synthetic aperture function is to force $t(x,y) = t_O(x,y) \cdot t_A(x,y)$ to become close to an MPF for *any* given complex object function $t_O(x,y)$. Once

$t(x, y) = t_O(x, y) \cdot t_A(x, y)$ is made close to an MPF (or even an exact MPF in some cases), the recovery of $t_O(x, y)$ from the two-dimensional FT magnitude of $t(x, y) = t_O(x, y) \cdot t_A(x, y)$ becomes quite easy, using either the analytical Hilbert transformation or the iterative error reduction algorithms discussed in earlier chapters.

Note that the effective system proposed in Fig. 1(b) is similar, at least in principle of operation, to a point-source FT holography system.[1] The recorded quantity is the same as in FT holography, i.e., the magnitude of the interference between the wavefronts generated from the hole region and the wavefronts generated from the object $t_O(x, y)$ is recorded in the spatial FT domain. However, the processing of the recorded FT magnitude in classical FT holography is similar to the analysis given in Chapter 3 regarding spectral interferometry. The proposed method of this chapter involves MPF based analysis of the recorded FT magnitude.

The required synthetic aperture can easily be fabricated by depositing a sub-micron thin metal layer (e.g., gold) onto a glass film, and leaving a small hole at the corner of the sample during the deposition process that precisely controls the overall field transmission of the sample. The shape of the hole is not critical; any shape will work. While the location of the hole on the synthetic aperture must be close to one of the corners, it does not matter which corner it is; using a different corner will simply flip the recovered complex image by 90° or 180° without changing any features. However, the size of the hole is critical. It must be sufficiently narrow that its spatial FT magnitude covers at least the maximum spatial frequency of the object image. In the ideal case, the hole should be as narrow as possible without violating the scalar field theory assumptions involved in all the imaging systems that yield FT magnitudes.[1] These assumptions require the hole size to be larger (by a factor of at least a few) than the wavelength of the probe light.

However, it is *totally incorrect* to conclude that the resolution of the recovered image is limited by the size of the hole. It was illustrated in Chapters 5 and 7 that a sample optical pulse (corresponding to the complex two-dimensional object function of this section) that is temporally only ~2-5 times as wide as the dummy strong pulse (corresponding to the 100% transmitting hole on the synthetic aperture) could be recovered with no resolution problems caused by the wide dummy pulse, i.e., the temporal resolution of the recovered sample pulse was much narrower than the temporal width of the dummy pulse.

Another important detail related to the choice of the hole size on the synthetic aperture is that, as has been described in Chapters 5 and 7, the recovery of the original image around the hole region will not be good. Actually the recovery around the hole region will be sacrificed for the excellent recovery of the remaining area on the object surface. Therefore, to loose as small an area as possible in the recovered image, choosing a small hole size in the synthetic aperture is also preferred. In fields, where information of the whole object image is required, two successive measurements with a different hole location in each measurement can be used to recover the whole object image without loss of information.

Finally, we would like to comment on the choice of the uniform transmission coefficient of the synthetic aperture. While a field transmission coefficient of ~30% or less generally works for SIMBA-based image recovery, choosing a very low transmission coefficient, e.g., less than or equal to ~1%, will degrade the noise performance of the technique. Ideally, as discussed in Chapters 5 and 7, the transmission coefficient of the synthetic aperture should be chosen just low enough that SIMBA converges, without reducing the noise performance of the technique.

9.2 FEMTOSECOND SPECTROSCOPY INVOLVING PUMP PROBE EXPERIMENTS

Femtosecond pulses have been extensively used in physics and chemistry[2-13] to resolve fast transient response of various material properties. What is typically measured is the transient changes induced in a material property due to the presence of a pump beam. Femtosecond spectral interferometry (SI) has been widely used to record these fast transient effects.[2-15]

While the set-up is quite different from one discipline to another, the pulse train shown in Fig. 2, composed of a reference pulse, followed in time by the pump pulse, which itself is followed by the probe pulse, is often a common factor. The function of the pump is simply to induce the transient change of interest in the material system. While the first reference pulse passes through the set-up without seeing the effect of the pump beam, the probe pulse picks up a certain phase and magnitude modulation due to the changes induced by the pump beam. This differential change in phase and magnitude of the probe pulse, as a function of time, is what carries the critical information on the transient response of the material of interest. This information is recorded by sending both the reference and the probe pulses collinearly to an optical spectrum analyzer, which measures the power spectrum of the pulse sequence, and therefore records the coherent interference of the two pulses in the frequency domain. The pump pulse is frequently filtered out of this pulse sequence prior to detection by choosing a different propagation direction.

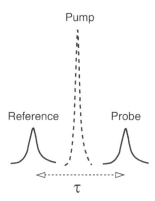

Fig. 2. Pulse train used in classical femtosecond spectroscopy.

Different approaches have been used in the past to recover the temporal phase and magnitude change induced by the pump pulse from a *single* power spectrum measurement of the above-mentioned pulse sequence. One important example is the FT based femtosecond spectroscopy, which takes a direct inverse FT (IFT) of the measured power spectrum of the pulse sequence.[5-15] However, this technique can only recover the *correlation* of the complex envelope function of the reference pulse with the probe pulse. The logistics of this approach are identical to the analytical techniques (described in the first half of Chapter 3) that were used to determine the nonlinearity profile of thin films.

In some fields, detecting the temporal correlation of the complex envelope function of the reference and probe pulses can be adequate. However in many other fields more information about the probe pulse is desired. In such cases, a self-referenced pulse characterization tool, such as frequency resolved optical gating[16] (FROG), can be used to uniquely characterize the reference pulse, and then the temporal profile of the probe pulse is fully retrieved from the correlation measurement.[10-13] The downside of this approach is the additional cost, complexity, and the longer measurement time associated with the complex FROG set-up.

In this section, we apply the same concepts of Spectral Interferometry using Minimum-phase Based Algorithms (SIMBA) described in Chapters 5 and 7 to the field of femtosecond spectroscopy. Rather taking a direct IFT of the measured power spectrum to recover the correlation function, we can actually apply the principles of SIMBA to recover the probe pulse profile. The only requirement is a dummy pulse to act as the reference pulse in Fig. 2. The new pulse train for SIMBA-based femtosecond spectroscopy is shown in Fig. 3. The restrictions on the dummy pulse properties are the same as described in Chapters 5 and 7, namely: (1) its bandwidth has to cover the bandwidth of the probe pulse; (2) its temporal width has to be narrower than the temporal width of the probe pulse, typically by a factor of ~5 or more; and (3) its peak amplitude has to be larger than the peak amplitude of the probe pulse, by a factor of ~5 or more. However, these three restrictions are quite loose. Actually, the first restriction on the bandwidth is not specific to SIMBA, and is shared by *all* the SI-based techniques. Furthermore, the third restriction can be an advantage, since it actually means that the higher power reference (dummy) pulse enhances the weak probe signal, as is well known heterodyne systems.[9]

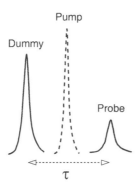

Fig. 3. Pulse train suggested for the SIMBA-based femtosecond spectroscopy.

The advantages of SIMBA-based femtosecond spectroscopy include: (1) no need for either a known reference pulse or a complex FROG set-up to measure the phase and magnitude of the reference pulse; (2) no minimum constraint on the delay parameter τ, which means that τ can be short and a lower resolution OSA can be used; (3) no time reversal ambiguity present (unlike second harmonic FROG); and (4) the signal-to-noise ratio is improved with respect to *all* SI-based techniques, because SIMBA makes use of the square root of the power spectrum rather than directly taking the IFT of the power spectrum itself. Actually, the second advantage mentioned above also allows the option to use the pump pulse as the reference (dummy) pulse itself, reducing by one the number of pulses used in the pulse train. This option will simplify the measurement set-up for certain applications that can work with a pump that is collinear with the probe pulse. The fact that the phase and magnitude of the pump pulse, which now acts as a dummy pulse as well, are modified by its interaction with the material system is not important for SIMBA-based femtosecond spectroscopy, as long as the above-mentioned restrictions on the dummy pump pulse are still met.

Finally, for practical issues related to spectral interferometry, we would like to recommend Refs. 14 and 15 as excellent sources of information. These references also discuss other fields, where our MPF-based approach could potentially be applied.

9.3 CHARACTERIZATION OF QUASI-PHASE MATCHED GRATINGS

This section will demonstrate the use of MPF based techniques to characterize the nonlinear coefficient profile of quasi-phase-matched (QPM) gratings. It is theoretically well known that, in a similar fashion to the Maker fringe analysis presented in Chapter 3, the measurement of the second-harmonic power generated by a QPM grating as a function of the frequency detuning parameter yields the Fourier transform (FT) *magnitude* of the *complex* nonlinear coefficient depth profile along the QPM device.[17] This FT magnitude spectrum measurement can be achieved by either tuning the wavelength of the fundamental laser beam or by tuning the temperature of the QPM grating (see Fig. 4).[17] In this section, we propose and demonstrate that from only this measurement of the FT magnitudes, recovery of the *period, envelope and chirp* parameters of a given QPM grating can be achieved using the same MPF based techniques described in earlier chapters.

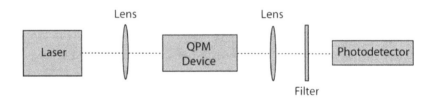

Fig. 4. QPM grating characterization set-up.

To expand the discussion, let us assume that for a QPM grating, the effective nonlinear coefficient profile along the grating can be generally written as:

$$d(z) = |d_o| \cdot \exp(j \cdot \Phi(z)) \cdot w(z/L - 1/2) \qquad (1)$$

where z is the position along the grating, $|d_o|$ is a scaling constant, L is the total length of the grating, and $w(z)$ is a windowing function that is usually estimated as $w(z) = rect(z)$, where $rect(z) = 1$ for $|z| < 1/2$ and 0 elsewhere. The phase term $\Phi(z)$ in Eq. (1) can take any functional form, depending on the design of the QPM grating. In this study we will analyze two special cases in detail:

(1) Uniform QPM gratings: $\Phi(z) = K_0 \cdot z = 2\pi/\Lambda_0 \cdot z$, where Λ_0 is the period of the QPM structure;

(2) Linearly chirped QPM gratings: $\Phi(z) = K_0 \cdot z + D_g \cdot z^2$.

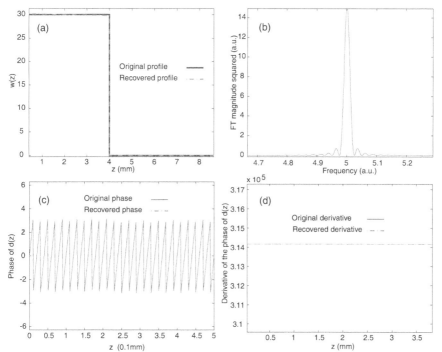

Fig. 5. (a) Envelope of the assumed uniform QPM grating; (b) theoretical frequency detuning curve of the same QPM grating; (b) phase of the nonlinear coefficient along the QPM device; and (d) derivative of the phase curve shown in (c), i.e., K_0. In (a), (c) and (d), the recovered quantities are shown with dashed curves; the theoretical curves are shown with solid lines.

For uniform gratings ($D_g = 0$), since $w(z)$ is *close* to an MPF, the iterative error-reduction algorithm (e.g., the Fienup algorithm) can be applied to the measured frequency detuning curve of a QPM grating to recover both K_0 and $w(z)$, given that $w(z)$

is *close* to an MPF. The numerical example shown in Fig. 5 demonstrates the recovery process for $w(z) = rect(z)$. Although $w(z) = rect(z)$ is not a *true* MPF, as discussed in Chapter 2, the recovery is excellent (see Fig. 5).

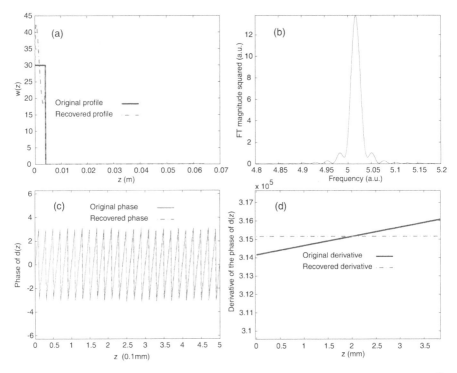

Fig. 6. Same as in Fig. 5, except for a linearly chirped QPM grating with $D_g = 0.25$ mm^{-2}.

For a linearly chirped grating ($D_g = 0.25$ mm^{-2} with $L = 4$ mm and a period of $\Lambda =$ 20 µm), as shown in Fig. 6, the recovery is not good for a windowing function choice of $w(z) = rect(z)$. In particular, the recovery of the windowing function $w(z)$ and of D_g is not acceptable (Figs. 6(a) and 6(d), respectively). This behavior is due to the fact that a linear phase chirp given with $\Phi(z) = K_0 \cdot z + D_g \cdot z^2$ pushes the overall nonlinearity profile given in Eq. (1) away from being close to an MPF.

However, by placing a thin QPM device with a stronger d coefficient (e.g., 30 pm/V) next to a weaker one (e.g., 10 pm/V) as shown in Fig. 7(a), the Fienup algorithm is forced to converge to the correct solution, even for a chirped grating. That is to say, $w(z)$ is forced to be close to an MPF, with a stronger peak at the origin ($z = 0$). The thickness of the stronger QPM device needs to be thinner than the QPM device of interest by ~3-5 times or more (see Fig. 7(a)). In this case, the recovery of both the phase $\Phi(z) = K_0 \cdot z + D_g \cdot z^2$ and its derivative is shown for $D_g = 0.25$ mm^{-2} in Fig. 7. The results reveal that the windowing function $w(z)$, K_0 and D_g of the QPM device can all be reliably recovered by using the Fienup algorithm for specially constructed devices, so that $w(z)$ exhibits a stronger peak close to the origin. The small glitches observed in the recovered derivative of the phase of $d(z)$ (Fig. 7(d)) are numerical artifacts, and can either be ignored or averaged out by low pass filtering.

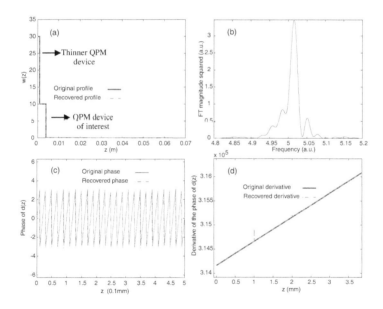

Fig. 7. Same as in Fig. 6, except that the chirped QPM grating is placed next to a stronger and thin device with a d coefficient of 30 pm/V.

9.4 CONCLUSIONS

This chapter has presented MPF-based solutions to three important problems . In the first problem, the complex transmission function of any planar object is recovered from only its two-dimensional FT magnitude using a synthetic aperture to manufacture an MPF. In the second problem, SIMBA-based femtosecond spectroscopy is discussed as a convenient alternative to existing techniques used to probe fast transient changes in different material systems. And in the final problem, MPF based characterization of QPM devices are illustrated. In our opinion, there are many other applications besides the examples treated in this thesis that can significantly benefit from MPF-based solutions; any physical problem, where an FT magnitude is measured, can potentially be treated with MPF based solutions. Our efforts in this thesis in general, and in this chapter in particular, simply point out the road to such breakthroughs.

REFERENCES

1. J. W. Goodman, Introduction to Fourier Optics, (Mc Graw-Hill, New York, 2002)

2. F. Reynaud, F. Salin, and A. Barthelemy, "Measurement of phase shifts introduced by nonlinear optical phenomena on subpicosecond pulses," Opt. Lett. 14, 275 (1989)

3. E. Tokunaga, A. Terasaki, and T. Kobayashi, "Frequency-domain interferometer for femtosecond time-resolved phase spectroscopy," Opt. Lett. 17, 1131 (1992)

4. E. Tokunaga, A. Terasaki, and T. Kobayashi, "Induced phase modulation of chirped continuum pulses studied with a femtosecond frequency-domain interferometer," Opt. Lett. 18, 370 (1993)

5. J. P. Geindre *et al.*, "Frequency-domain interferometer for measuring the phase and amplitude of a femtosecond pulse probing a laser-produced plasma," Opt. Lett. 19, 1997 (1994)

6. C. W. Siders *et al.*, "Plasma-based accelerator diagnostics based upon longitudinal interferometry with ultrashort optical pulses," IEEE Trans. Plasma Science 24, 301 (1996)

7. C. W. Siders *et al.*, "Laser wakefield excitation and measurement by femtosecond longitudinal interferometry," Phys. Rev. Lett. 76, 3570 (1996)

8. R. Zgadzaj, et al., "Femtosecond pump-probe study of preformed plasma channels," J. Opt. Soc. Am. B 21, 1559 (2004)

9. L. Lepetit, G. Cheriaux, and M. Joffre, "Linear techniques of phase measurement by femtosecond spectral interferometry for applications in spectroscopy," J. Opt. Soc. Am. B 12, 2467 (1995)

10. S. M. Ghallager, et al., "Heterodyne detection of the complete electric field of femtosecond four-wave mixing signals," J. Opt. Soc. Am. B 15, 2338 (1998)

11. J. Tignon, M. V. Marquezini, T. Hasche, and D. S. Chemla, "Spectral interferometry of semiconductor nanostructures," IEEE J. Quantum Electron. 35, 510 (1999)

12. X. Chen, *et al.*, "Temporally and spectrally resolved amplitude and phase of coherent four-wave-mixing emission from GaAs quantum wells," Phys. Rev. B 56, 9738 (1997)

13. D. Birkedal, and J. Shah, "Femtosecond spectral interferometry of resonant secondary emission from quantum wells: Resonance Rayleigh scattering in the nonergodic regime," Phys. Rev. Lett. 81, 2372 (1998)

14. C. Dorrer, N. Belabas, J.P. Likforman, and M. Joffre, "Spectral resolution and sampling issues in Fourier-transform spectral interferometry," J. Opt. Soc. Am. B 17, 1795 (2000)

15. C. Dorrer, "Influence of the calibration of the detector on spectral interferometry," J. Opt. Soc. Am. B 16, 1160 (1999)

16. R. Trebino, and D. J. Kane, "Using phase retrieval to measure the intensity and phase of ultrashort pulses: frequency-resolved optical gating", J. Opt. Soc. Am. A 10, 1101, (1993)

17. G. Imeshev, "Tailoring of ultrafast frequency conversion with quasi-phase-matching gratings," Ph.D. dissertation submitted to the Department of Applied Physics, Stanford University, Stanford, CA (2000)

CHAPTER 10: CONCLUSIONS

To laugh often and much;
To win the respect of intelligent people and the affection of children;
To earn the appreciation of honest critics and endure the betrayal of false friends;
To appreciate beauty, to find the best in others;
To leave the world a bit better...
To know even one life has breathed easier because you have lived.
This is to have succeeded.
Ralph Waldo Emerson

In this dissertation, we have introduced various nondestructive characterization tools to uniquely recover the Fourier transform phase of a function of interest from a Fourier transform magnitude measurement. The unique FT phase recovery allowed us to characterize the target function in various fields using a single inverse Fourier transform operation. Our techniques can be grouped into two categories: (1) non-interferometric techniques; and (2) interferometric techniques.

In the first category, the measurement of the FT magnitude of the target function *alone* is used to recover its FT phase uniquely. The recovery algorithm is based on the property of a special class of functions known as minimum phase functions (MPF); MPFs make it possible to uniquely relate the FT phase to the FT magnitude, either analytically using the logarithmic Hilbert transformation, or iteratively. We have shown through both numerical simulations and experiments that an iterative recovery technique, based on error-reduction algorithms such as the Fienup algorithm, works very well for the characterization of nonlinear thin films (Chapters 3-4) and fiber Bragg gratings (Chapter 6). As a result of this work, the second-order nonlinearity profile of poled silica samples were recovered uniquely, for the first time, a challenging task that was not possible before these techniques were developed. This enabled us to learn more about the physics of the induced nonlinearity in poled glasses and as a result to optimize the peak nonlinear coefficient in thermally poled germanosilicate thin films to yield a record high nonlinearity of 1.6 pm/V. In the area of fiber Bragg gratings, this concept led to the recovery of the group delay spectra using only magnitude spectrum measurements. This simple yet powerful approach is potentially an important alternative to expensive test equipment such as network analyzers currently used in the industry.

Our interferometric techniques can be divided into two sub-categories: (1) the classical spectral interferometry (SI) technique; and (2) the minimum-phase based spectral interferometry technique, i.e., SIMBA. In the first half of Chapter 3, we demonstrated powerful versions of the classical SI technique to uniquely characterize nonlinear thin films. Starting with Chapter 5, we discussed various advantages of the powerful SIMBA technique with respect to the classical SI, such as better noise performance, simplicity and convenience (since it does not depend on an already characterized reference function), the flexibility to use a lower resolution spectrum analyzer, etc. In Chapters 5,7-9, several applications of the powerful SIMBA are introduced: ultrashort pulse characterization, fiber Bragg grating characterization, optical coherence tomography, optical image processing, and femtosecond spectroscopy.

In future work, we plan to expand the powerful SIMBA technique to other fields that are currently using classical SI techniques. Because of its flexibility, SIMBA also opens up the possibility of solving other problems, where a classical SI approach cannot be applied, and creating new applications in which SI has never been tried. Furthermore, with the development of better initial condition estimation, convergence of the iterative phase recovery could be sped up by an order of magnitude. Finally, the application of the wavelet analysis tools to improve SIMBA is another direction yet to be examined.

APPENDIX A: THE TWIN SAMPLE AND THE REFERENCE SAMPLE METHODS

> *Everything should be made as simple as possible, but not simpler.*
> *Albert Einstein*

In this appendix, two special cases of the general theory (the two-sample technique) introduced in Section 3.1.2 of Chapter 3 to recover the second-order optical nonlinearity depth profiles of thin films is discussed.

A.1 TWIN-SAMPLE METHOD

In this sub-section of Appendix A, we treat a first special case of the two-sample technique, namely the situation where nonlinear samples A and B have the same profile, $d_A(z) = d_B(z)$. This occurs, for example, when the samples are two pieces cut from the same sample. This configuration is of interest because it requires only a single sample, thus, measurements are simplified. This is referred to as the twin-sample method.[1]

A.1.1 FIRST SOLUTION

The special case $d_A(z) = d_B(z)$ can, of course, always be solved using the general treatment presented in Section 3.1.2 of Chapter 3. However, there is a simpler solution. Since the number of unknown samples is reduced from two to one, we expect intuitively that it should be possible to recover $d_A(z)$ completely from a single MF curve, for example $MF_{S1}(f)$. This line of reasoning can be better understood by recognizing that since $d_A(z) = d_B(z)$, it follows that $MF_A = MF_B$, $|D_A| = |D_B|$, and $\phi_A = \phi_B$. Equation (5) of Chapter 3 then shows that $MF_{S2} = 2|D_A|^2(1 + \cos\phi_2)$ is now independent of ϕ_A, so the MF curve of S2 configuration (see Fig. 4 of Chapter 3) does not contain any FT phase information and no longer needs to be measured. The key to the recovery of ϕ_A is now entirely contained in the MF curve of sandwich S1. Indeed, inserting the above equalities in Eq. (4) of Chapter 3 yields the following expression for this curve:

$$MF_{S1} = |D_{S1}|^2 = 2|D_A|^2 - 2|D_A|^2 \cos(2\phi_A + \phi_1) \qquad (A1)$$

To illustrate how $d_A(z)$ (and thus $d_B(z)$ as well) is recovered from this MF curve alone, we use the arbitrary exemplary profile shown in Fig. A1(a) and assume $L_{GI} = 52\ \mu m$. The calculated MF curve of the sandwich S1 that is formed by clamping this sample against itself is shown in Fig. A1(b).

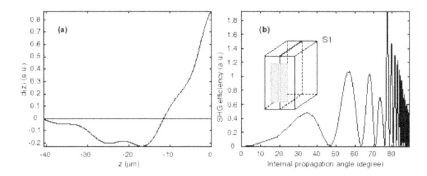

Fig. A1. (a) Arbitrarily chosen nonlinearity profile to verify the twin-sample technique, (b) MF curve for the S1 configuration in the twin-sample method, calculated numerically by using the profile given in (a).

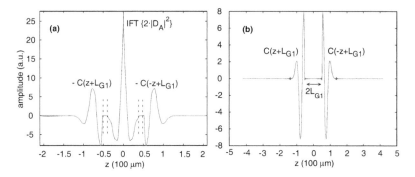

Fig. A2. (a) IFT of MF_{S1}, (b) IFT of $-\left|D_{S1}\right|^2 + 2\left|D_A\right|^2$.

The first step in the recovery is to take the IFT of MF_{S1}, which gives:

$$IFT\{MF_{S1}\} = IFT\left\{\left|D_A\right|^2\right\} - IFT\left\{\left|D_A\right|^2 \cos(2\phi_A + \phi_1)\right\} \qquad (A2)$$

218

This IFT is plotted in Fig. A2(a). It is composed of two terms, $IFT\left\{|D_A|^2\right\}$ and $IFT\left\{|D_A|^2\cos(2\phi_A+\phi_1)\right\}$. The first term is proportional to the auto-correlation function of $d_A(z)$, and, as mentioned in Chapter 3, it can provide the depth but not the functional form of the nonlinear region. The second term is the one that contains both the FT phase and FT amplitude information. It can be expanded as:

$$IFT\left\{|D_A|^2\cos(2\phi_A+\phi_1)\right\}=C(z+L_{G1})+C(-z+L_{G1}) \qquad (A3)$$

where $C(z)=d_A(z)*d_A(z)$ is the auto-convolution of $d_A(z)$. These two terms are identified in Fig. A2(a). It can be shown that if $L_{G1}>W$, where $W=W_A=W_B$ is the depth of the nonlinear region, then $C(z+L_{G1})$, $C(-z+L_{G1})$, and $IFT\left\{|D_A|^2\right\}$ do not overlap. The second step of the algorithm is to recover $C(z+L_{G1})$ from $IFT\{MF_{S1}\}$, which determines $C(z)$. The FT of $C(z)$ is equal to $|D_A|^2\exp(j2\phi_A)$, which is the square of the FT of $d_A(z)$. The last step is to take the IFT of the square root of $|D_A|^2\exp(j2\phi_A)$ to obtain $d_A(z)=d_B(z)$.

As before, the condition $L_{G1}>W$ required for this technique to work can always be satisfied in practice by using a thick enough spacer in sandwich structure S1. However, for situations where meeting this condition is difficult, Eq. (A1) can still be solved by making use of additional information, namely the measured MF curve of sample A, alone. The process is then much the same as in the two-sample technique, namely we now take the IFT of the linear combination $-|D_{S1}|^2+2|D_A|^2$, which is:

$$IFT\left\{-|D_{S1}|^2+2|D_A|^2\right\}=IFT\left\{|D_A|^2\cos(2\phi_A+\phi_1)\right\}=C(z+L_{G1})+C(-z+L_{G1}) \quad (A4)$$

This IFT is plotted in Fig. A2(b). The two convolution terms in Eq. (A4) never overlap spatially, so from this IFT, the convolution function $C(z+L_{G1})$ and hence $C(z)$ are easily recovered. The rest of the recovery process is identical to the $L_{G1}>W$ case.

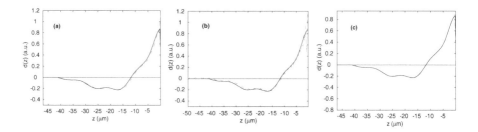

Fig. A3. Result of the recovery (dashed curves) for the twin-sample method using (a) the first solution, (b) the second solution; (c) result of the recovery (dashed curve) for the reference-sample method. The solid curves represent the theoretically assumed nonlinearity profiles. In (c) the recovered profile is essentially indistinguishable from the original profile, except near z = 0.

The profile recovered by this method is plotted in Fig. A3(a) (dashed curve), together with the actual profile (solid curve) taken from Fig. A1(a). Again, the recovery is very good, with an average error of only 0.71%.

A.1.2 SECOND SOLUTION

While this alternative solution to solving the $d_A(z) = d_B(z)$ case is computationally more challenging, it offers an important insight into the problem. We start by rewriting Eq. (A1) in the form:

$$MF_{S1} = 2|D_A|^2 (1 - \cos(2\phi_A + \phi_1)) = 4|D_A|^2 \sin^2(\phi_A + \frac{\phi_1}{2}) \qquad (A5)$$

This expression is the square of the magnitude of the Hartley transform (HT) of $d_{S1}(z)$. Since $d_{S1}(z)$ is a real and odd function of z, the relationship between the FT and HT of $d_{S1}(z)$ is simply $H(f) = jF(f)$, where H and F denote the HT and the FT, respectively. Therefore, the MF measurement of S1 provides the magnitude of the Hartley transform of $d_{S1}(z) = d_A(z) - d_A(-z + L_{G1})$. Since $d_{S1}(z)$ is real, so is its HT, which means that the phase of the HT can only take values of 0 or π. Because of this important property, knowledge of the HT magnitude is sufficient to uniquely recover a real function.[2] Several algorithms have been developed to achieve such a recovery.[2-4] Since $d_{S1}(z)$ is a real and odd function, all algorithms require only half of the frequency spectrum. The recovered profile $d_{S1}(z)$ is also an odd function, and either its $z < 0$ or $z > 0$ portion is equal to the nonlinearity profile $d_A(z) = d_B(z)$.

Application of this principle yields the recovered profile shown in Fig. A3(b). Again, the recovered profile is very close to the original one. The average error resulting from this recovery process is ~4.4%. This comparatively lower performance compared to previous methods is believed to be due to the algorithm used to recover the HT of a real function from its HT magnitude.

A.2 THE REFERENCE-SAMPLE METHOD

This is perhaps the most useful of the three IFT techniques. The basic concept is to use an already characterized reference sample with a known nonlinearity profile $d_R(z)$ to determine the profile $d_U(z)$ of an unknown sample.[5] Once again, since the number of unknown profiles is reduced to one, we expect that a single MF measurement should be sufficient, as we show below. Besides a reduced number of measurements, this method offers several significant advantages, including a faster recovery process, simpler coding of the recovery algorithm, and the ability to recover the sign of $d(z)$ if the reference nonlinearity profile has a known sign.

In practice, a thin wafer of LiNbO$_3$, KDP, or another nonlinear material of known thickness can serve as the reference sample. Since their nonlinearity profile is in principle a simple rectangular function, just knowing the thickness of the crystal would be sufficient. A poled silica sample that has been reliably characterized by any of the above methods can also serve as a reference sample. However, one needs to use a reference that has a similar refractive index to that of the sample to be characterized. This will avoid complications arising from refractive index mismatch between the samples, which becomes quite dominant especially at high internal propagation angles.

Once again, with this method the magnitude and the phase of the FT of the unknown sample's nonlinearity profile $d_U(z)$ are obtained from the single measurement of the MF curve of the sandwich structure formed by mating this sample with the reference sample of a known profile $d_R(z)$. These samples can be mated in four possible configurations, depending on which of their two surfaces are in contact. In principle, each of these four configurations can be used to recover $d_U(z)$. Since the recovery process is similar for all four configurations, we will only illustrate it here for the S2 configuration. The effective nonlinearity profile of S2 can be written as $d_{S2}(z) = d_U(z) + d_R(z - L)$, where $L = L_{G2} + L_R$, L_R is the total thickness of the reference sample, and L_{G2} the separation between the two samples. The MF curve of S2 is given by Eq. (5) of Chapter 3:

$$MF_{S2} = |D_{S2}|^2 = |D_R|^2 + |D_U|^2 + 2|D_R||D_U|\cos(\phi_U - \phi_R + \phi) \qquad (A6)$$

where $|D_R|$, $|D_U|$, ϕ_R, and ϕ_U are the FT magnitudes and phases of $d_R(z)$ and $d_U(z)$, respectively, and $\phi(f) = 2\pi f L$. To simulate this technique, we use the same two nonlinearity profiles as before, shown in Fig. 3(a) of Chapter 3, with $L = 190$ μm and $L_{G1} = L_{G2} = 40$ μm. The profile of sample B is taken to be the known reference profile and the profile of sample A is assumed to be the unknown profile. The MF curve of S2 computed with these assumptions is the same as the curve shown previously in Fig. 4(d) of Chapter 3.

The algorithm used to retrieve the unknown profile is similar to the algorithms described in the previous sections and can be summarized as follows. The first step is to take the IFT of $|D_{S2}|^2$, i.e.:

$$IFT\left\{|D_{S2}|^2\right\} = IFT\left\{|D_R|^2 + |D_U|^2\right\} + IFT\left\{2|D_R||D_U|\cos(\phi_U - \phi_R + \phi)\right\} \qquad (A7)$$

The second IFT term in Eq. (A7) can be written as the sum $C(z + L) + C(-z + L)$, where $C(z) = d_U(z) * d_R(-z)$. By choosing a sufficiently thick reference sample, i.e., $L > W_R + \max\{W_U, W_R\}$, where W_U and W_R are the depths of $d_U(z)$ and $d_R(z)$, respectively, $C(z + L)$, $C(-z + L)$, and $IFT\left\{|D_R|^2 + |D_U|^2\right\}$ do not spatially overlap. The second step is to recover either $C(z + L)$ or $C(-z + L)$), which yields $C(z)$. In the third step, we calculate the FT of $C(z)$, which is equal to $|D_U||D_R|\exp(j(\phi_U - \phi_R))$. Since the reference nonlinearity profile $d_R(z)$ is known, both $|D_U|$ and ϕ_U are easily recovered from this FT. This constitutes the main difference with, and improvement over the two-sample and twin-sample techniques. The last step is to take the IFT of the recovered Fourier transform $|D_U| \exp(j\phi_U)$ to obtain the unknown profile $d_U(z)$.

If the condition $L > W_R + \max\{W_U, W_R\}$ is difficult to satisfy, the MF curve of the unknown sample can be measured (as in the previous methods), and $IFT\{|D_{S2}|^2 - |D_R|^2 - |D_U|^2\} = IFT\{2|D_R||D_U|\cos(\phi_U - \phi_R + \phi)\}$ can be calculated to recover $C(z)$ without spatial overlapping. The main difference is that the MF curve of the reference sample no longer needs to be measured, since it can be computed numerically from the known reference profile. The rest of the recovery process is the same as described in the earlier sections.

The comparison of the recovered unknown profile with the original profile is shown in Fig. A3(c). The recovery is excellent, except within ~1 μm of $z = 0$. The average error in the recovered profile is 1%. Most of this error comes from the discrepancy in the interval -1 μm $< z <$ 0. The error in the rest of the profile ($z <$ -1 μm) is in fact remarkably low (0.01%).

All numerical simulations presented in this appendix and in Section 3.1.2 of Chapter 3 used 2048 data points in the Fourier transforms. In all three techniques, application of the Papoulis-Gerchberg (PG) algorithm[6-8] is the most time-consuming portion of the code. For the reference-sample and twin-sample techniques, since only one MF measurement is required, the PG algorithm is applied to a single MF measurement, which takes ~5 minutes with a 500 MHz computer. For the two-sample technique, at least two MF measurements are required and the PG algorithm running time at least doubles (~10 minutes). The remaining portions of the computer codes are very similar for all three techniques, and the rest of the running time is less than ~10 s. The only exception is the second solution of the twin-sample technique, involving Hartley transforms, which is considerably slower and typically takes 1–2 hours for the same accuracy levels.

REFERENCES

1. A. Ozcan, M. J. F. Digonnet, G. S. Kino, "Inverse Fourier transform technique to determine second-order optical nonlinearity spatial profiles," Appl. Phys. Lett. 82, 1362, (2003)

2. N. Nakajima, "Reconstruction of a real function from its Hartley-transform intensity," J. Opt. Soc. Am. A 5, 858 (1988)

3. G. S. Chen, J. L. Wu, L. S. Lee, "Signal extrapolation from Hartley transform magnitudes," Electron. Lett. 26, 793 (1990)

4. R. P. Millane, "Analytical properties of the Hartley transform and their implications," Proc. IEEE 82, 413 (1994)

5. A. Ozcan, M. J. F. Digonnet, and G. S. Kino, "Simplified inverse Fourier transform technique to measure optical nonlinearity profiles using reference sample," Electron. Lett. 40, 551, (2004)

6. P. J. S. G. Ferreira, "Interpolation and the discrete Papoulis-Gerchberg algorithm," IEEE Trans. on Signal Processing 42, 2596 (1994)

7. A. Papoulis, "New algorithm in spectral analysis and band-limited extrapolation," IEEE Trans. Circuits, Syst. 22, 735 (1975)

8. R. W. Gerchberg, "Super-resolution through error energy reduction," Opt. Acta. 21, 709 (1974)

APPENDIX B: PAPOULIS-GERCHBERG (PG) ALGORITHM

It is well known that, in principle, the full Fourier transform spectrum of an *entire* function can be reconstructed from the sole knowledge of limited portions of this spectrum.[1-5] This is accomplished by using the principle of analytic continuation, i.e., by extrapolating the FT from its known frequency intervals into the unknown intervals, using either analytical or iterative methods.[1-3] To illustrate this principle in the particular context of measured Maker fringes, we assume, without loss of generality, that the nonlinearity spatial profile $d(z)$ is bounded between $z = -W$ and $z = 0$, where W, a positive quantity, is the depth of the nonlinear region; outside this region $d(z) = 0$. This definition implies that the convolution function $C(z)$ is zero for $|z| > W$. Note that, as pointed out in Chapter 3, $IFT\left\{ \left| D(f) \right|^2 \right\} = C(z) = d(z) \otimes d(z) = d(z) * d(-z)$, where '$\otimes$' and '$*$' stand for the correlation and convolution operations, respectively. In other words, $d(z)$ and hence $C(z)$ are space-limited functions, i.e., they are zero outside some finite region. The Fourier transforms of such functions are known to be entire functions, i.e., analytical over the entire complex domain.[4] Therefore, $D(f)$ and $\left| D(f) \right|^2$ are both entire functions, and in principle, knowing their values in only a limited frequency interval is enough to uniquely retrieve the whole frequency spectrum by using the principle of analytic continuation.[4-5] However, we cannot apply this principle of analytic continuation to $D(f)$, even though it is an entire function, because we only know $\left| D(f) \right|$ and the phase information of $D(f)$ is not available. However, for $\left| D(f) \right|^2$, which is also an entire function, we do not need the phase information to apply this principle and we already know $\left| D(f) \right|^2$ in the intervals $[-f_{max}, -f_{min}]$ and $[f_{min}, f_{max}]$ (see Chapter 3). What is more important is that since $\left| D(f) \right|^2$ is a real and non-negative quantity for all f, which makes the application of the analytical continuation principle to $\left| D(f) \right|^2$ much easier and more robust, than its application to $D(f)$, which is in general a complex quantity.

The Papoulis-Gerchberg (PG) algorithm[1,6,7] is one of the most common iterative methods used for analytic continuation. How the PG iterative process is applied to the Maker fringe (MF) analysis, is summarized in Fig. B1. In the first step, zeros are inserted for all the unmeasured values of $|D(f)|^2$. Next, the IFT of $|D(f)|^2$ is computed to obtain a first estimate $C'(z)$ of $C(z)$. We then preserve only the *real* part of $C'(z)$ and replace all the points of $C'(z)$ outside the $|z| < W$ region with zeros. Then the FT of this new function is taken, which yields $C''(f)$. By taking the real part and then the absolute value of $C''(f)$, a new estimate $|D(f)|^2_{new}$ of $|D(f)|^2$ is obtained. The measured values of $|D(f)|^2$ in the frequency intervals $[-f_{max}, -f_{min}]$ and $[f_{min}, f_{max}]$ are retained, and in the rest of the frequency spectrum the unmeasured values, which were set to zero in the first step, are replaced by the corresponding values of $|D(f)|^2_{new}$. The IFT of this new function is calculated to obtain a second estimate $C'(z)$ of $C(z)$. The above steps are repeated on $C'(z)$ until the change in two successive estimates of $|D(f)|^2$ is negligible.

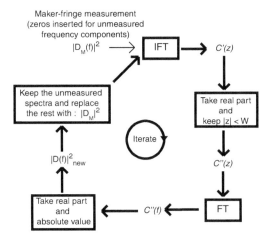

Fig. B1. Flow chart showing the details of the iterative PG algorithm.

The convergence rate of this algorithm depends on how well the depth W of $d(z)$ is known. For nonlinear materials such as LiNbO$_3$ or KDP, W can be measured very accurately. For poled silica, it can be estimated by somewhat less accurate means, for example by etching techniques[8] or by scanning the nonlinear region with a tightly focused fundamental beam. However, these measurements are not necessary because the PG algorithm itself can provide a good estimate of W. To do so, we start with an initial estimate of W, e.g., $W = dW$, where dW is the resolution required for W, and apply the PG algorithm. The algorithm provides an estimate for $C(z)$. We then calculate the percentage

of $|C(z)|$ contained in the $|z| < W$ region, which is equal to $\rho = \int\limits_{-W}^{W} |C(z)| dz \Big/ \int\limits_{-\infty}^{\infty} |C(z)| dz$.

The initial estimate of W is then increased by dW, and this computation is repeated for this new value. The correct value of W is attained when $\rho = 1$. In practice the depth is accurate enough and this iterative process can be terminated when $\rho > 99.99\%$ if the data is clean, or at a lower value (e.g., $\rho = 98\%$) in the presence of noise.

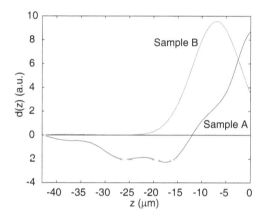

Fig. B2. Arbitrarily chosen nonlinearity profiles to apply the PG algorithm for sample A and sample B.

Simulations of both the recovery of W and extrapolation of the missing portions of $|D(f)|^2$ are illustrated with a numerical example. Fig. B2 shows two arbitrarily chosen nonlinearity profiles for samples A and B. The respective depths of these profiles are $W_A = 42.66 \mu m$ and $W_B \approx 24 \mu m$. Application of the above algorithm to estimate W for both samples yielded $W_A = 42.37 \mu m$ and $W_B = 22.98 \mu m$, when the algorithm was stopped at $\rho = 99.95\%$. The error in the recovered depth is ~0.7 % for sample A and ~4.25 % for sample B. The relatively poor performance for sample B occurs primarily because sample

B's profile is a slowly decaying function, which means that a minor fraction of the profile lies in the range 22.98 µm $< z <$ 24 µm. A more accurate value of W_B can be recovered by increasing the convergence value for ρ. For example with $\rho = 99.99$ % we obtain a recovered depth $W_B = 23.81$ µm, or an error of only ~0.7%.

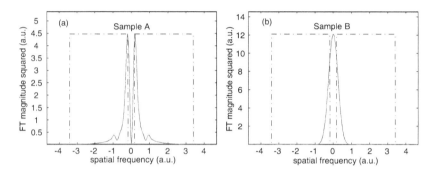

Fig. B3. (a), (b) Square of the magnitude of the FT spectrum (both the theoretical and the recovered spectra are superimposed) of the nonlinearity profiles of sample A and sample B, respectively. The dashed rectangular curves denote the frequency range that the MF measurements provide.

However, accurate knowledge of W_B is not necessary for the PG algorithm to work well; to prove this point, we will implement it in the following example with the less accurate of the two width values ($W_B = 22.98$ µm) Figures A3(a) and A3(b) show the full theoretical FT of the nonlinearity profiles of samples A and B, respectively. The figures also show the corresponding full FT spectrum, recovered using the PG algorithm. In each figure, the portions of the spectra within the dashed rectangles represent the frequency ranges $[-f_{max}, -f_{min}]$ and $[f_{min}, f_{max}]$ over which the FT spectra would have been known had we obtained these spectra by an MF measurement. The portions of the FT spectra outside of these rectangles are the portions recovered by application of the PG algorithm. It is clear that the recovery is excellent, i.e., the theoretical and recovered FT spectra for both of the samples are so close that they are indistinguishable. The difference between the exact and recovered spectra defined as $\dfrac{\int \left(|D(f)| - |\hat{D}(f)| \right)^2 df}{\int |D(f)|^2 df}$, where $|\hat{D}(f)|$

is an estimate of $|D(f)|$, is less than ~0.043% for sample A and ~0.078% for sample B.

The application of the PG algorithm to estimate the missing parts in the spectrum of $MF_{S2}(f)$ (see Chapter 3) is slightly different from estimating the unknown frequencies for $MF_A(f)$ and $MF_B(f)$. In the latter, all the points of $C'(z)$, i.e., the first estimate of $IFT\{|D(f)|^2\}$, outside the $|z| < W$ region are replaced with zeros, and the FT of this new function is taken to obtain a new estimate for $|D(f)|^2$, i.e., $|D(f)|^2_{new}$ (see Fig. B1). However, for $MF_{S2}(f) = |D_{S2}(f)|^2$, if $L > W_B + \max\{W_A, W_B\}$, then there is an important extra piece of information available to improve the convergence of the algorithm shown in Fig. B1: namely, $IFT\{|D_{S2}(f)|^2\} = C'(z)$ is known to be zero in the regions $|z| > L + W_A$ and $\max\{W_A, W_B\} < |z| < L - W_B$. Therefore, in the PG algorithm shown in Fig. B1, at every iteration $C'(z)$ can be replaced with zeros in the regions just mentioned. This same principle can also be applied for $MF_{S1}(f) = |D_{S1}(f)|^2$. If $L_{G1} > \max\{W_A, W_B\}$, then for $IFT\{|D_{S1}(f)|^2\} = C'(z)$, the regions $|z| > L_{G1} + W_A + W_B$ and $\max\{W_A, W_B\} < |z| < L_{G1}$ are known to be zero. This additional information can be used in the PG algorithm to improve the speed of the convergence and the accuracy of the recovery for a given number of iterations.

REFERENCES

1. P. J. S. G. Ferreira, "Interpolation and the discrete Papoulis-Gerchberg algorithm," IEEE Trans. on Signal Processing 42, 2596 (1994)

2. M. Soumekh, "Band-limited interpolation from unevenly spaced sampled data," IEEE Trans. on Acoustics, Speech and Signal Processing 36, 110 (1988)

3. D. J. Wingham, "The reconstruction of a band-limited function and its Fourier transform from a finite number of samples at arbitrary locations by singular value decomposition," IEEE Trans. on Signal Processing 40, 559 (1992)

4. Y. Katznelson, in *An introduction to Harmonic Analysis*, (Dover Publications, New York, 1976)

5. K. R. Castleman, in *Digital Image Processing*, (Prentice Hall, New Jersey, 1979)

6. A. Papoulis, "New algorithm in spectral analysis and band-limited extrapolation," IEEE Trans. Circuits, Syst. 22, 735 (1975)

7. R. W. Gerchberg, "Super-resolution through error energy reduction," Opt. Acta. 21, 709 (1974)

8. A. L. C. Triques, C. M. B. Cordeiro, V. Balestrieri, B. Lesche, W. Margulis, and I. C. S Carvalho, "Depletion region in thermally poled fused silica, "Appl. Phys. Lett. 76, 2496 (2000)

APPENDIX C: ADVANTAGES OF CYLINDER ASSISTED MAKER FRINGE TECHNIQUE

For all of the analytical and iterative Fourier transform (FT) techniques discussed in Chapter 3 to be accurate, it is essential to measure the FT of the nonlinearity profile up to the highest possible spatial frequency, f. Since to a first order approximation, f is proportional to $|1/\cos\theta|$, where θ is the internal propagation angle inside the nonlinear crystal, it is quite important to measure Maker fringe (MF) curves[1] up to as close to the maximum incidence angle (90°) as possible. This is especially important for thin nonlinear regions (a few microns), since the FT spectrum is broad for thin samples, and most of the information is contained in the high-frequency region. However, in an MF measurement, the maximum achievable angle is strongly limited by total internal reflection (TIR) at the output face of the sample: above this angle, the SH signal is totally reflected at the air-sample interface and does not reach the detector. This limitation can be quite serious: for example, for poled silica the TIR angle is as low as $\theta_{max} \approx 43°$. Two methods have been developed to overcome TIR, namely the prism-assisted MFT (PMFT)[2] and the sphere-assisted MFT (SMFT)[3]. In PMFT, a prism made of the same material as the nonlinear sample is clamped against each of the two sides of the sample, avoiding TIR at both interfaces.[2] The laser is injected into the sample through one prism, and the SH is collected through the other. The input prism eliminates Fresnel reflection loss, which is sizable at high incidence angles, and the output prism eliminates TIR at the output face. In SMFT, the same functions are achieved with two half-spheres.[3] In both techniques, a thin layer of index-matching gel or liquid is placed between the sample and the prism or half-sphere to avoid TIR and optical losses at these interfaces.

In this appendix, we describe an additional improvement to these techniques that utilizes half-cylinders [4] instead of prisms or half-spheres. The nonlinear sample is sandwiched between two half-cylinders made of the same material as the sample, as illustrated in Fig. C1. The laser beam is focused with a spherical lens, and launched into the nonlinear sample through the input half-cylinder, and the SH beam generated by the sample is collected through the output half-cylinder. The distance L between the lens and the input half-cylinder (see Fig. C1(b)) is adjusted so that the laser beam is focused on the input face of the sample. Because it is focused by a half-cylinder, the laser beam is actually focused in different planes in the x and y directions, as defined in Fig. C1(a); however, this difference is slight, as will be discussed below. This cylinder-assisted MF technique (CMFT) offers several decisive advantages over existing techniques, which allowed us to measure Maker fringes up to a record high internal propagation angle of 89.6°.[4] Consequently, the CMFT is especially well suited to determine the nonlinearity profile of thin samples using FT techniques described in Chapter 3.

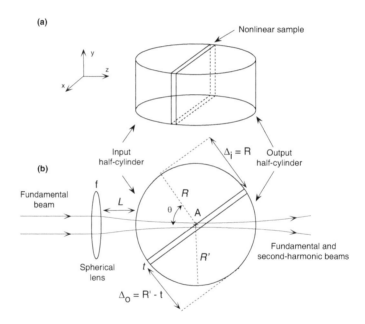

Fig. C1 (a) Diagram of the test nonlinear sample placed between two half-cylinders. (b) Top view of the sample/half-cylinders assembly, and of the spherical lens used to focus the beam through the input half-cylinder.

C.1 ADVANTAGES OF CMFT OVER PMFT

The CMFT[4] presents a number of advantages over the PMFT[2], some of which are also shared by the SMFT, as described in Ref. 3. First, after the incident laser beam has been aligned so that it is incident on the input half-cylinder at normal incidence, this incidence remains normal for any angle θ, as can be readily seen in Fig. C1(b). In other words, as the sample is rotated from $\theta = 0°$ to $\theta = 90°$, the laser beam is always incident on the same point on the sample (point A in Fig. C1(b)), i.e., it is always the same point on the sample that is being probed. This advantage is particularly important when the nonlinearity profile is not completely homogeneous across the face of the sample, in which case probing different points would impair the accuracy of the MF curve and thus the accuracy of the inferred nonlinearity profile. In order for the laser to be incident on the same point, the longitudinal axis of the input half-cylinder must be exactly *on* the input face of the sample, as illustrated in Fig. C1(b). This condition is satisfied, provided the input half-cylinder is a true half-cylinder, i.e., a cylinder cut to a thickness Δ_i equal to its radius R (see Fig. C1(b)). In contrast, using the prism-assisted technique, the input beam is steered as the sample is rotated (see Fig. C2); thus, it is impossible to examine the same point without realigning the sample with respect to the laser beam for each incidence angle. This requirement increases measurement time, and since it is difficult to identify point A in practice, the correction is never complete and measurement uncertainties are introduced. Furthermore, to probe incidence angles covering a sizable fraction of the full range requires the use of prisms with different angles, for example one prism for low angles and one for high angles, which again complicates measurements and introduces errors.

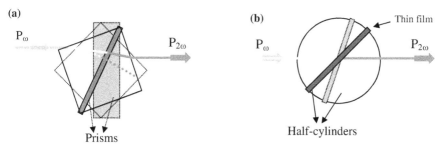

Fig. C2 Illustration of beam steering occurring for (a) PMFT and its comparison with (b) CMFT.

Second, because the laser beam is always incident on the input half-cylinder at 90°, the Fresnel reflection loss at this interface is as small as possible, and most important, it is independent of incidence angle. Thus, any possible error in the calibration of the Fresnel loss of the laser beam at this interface is significantly reduced. Similarly, the output SH beam crosses the output face of the output half-cylinder at normal incidence for any value of the incidence angle θ, thus, the Fresnel loss experienced by the SH beam is again small and independent of θ. For this property to hold, i.e., for the SH beam to be normally incident on the output half-cylinder at all angles, the distance traveled by the SH beam between point A (its point of origin, see Fig. C1(b)) and the output face of the output half-cylinder must be independent of θ. Consequently, as illustrated in Fig. C1(b), the thickness of the output half-cylinder must be equal to $\Delta_o = R'$ – t, where R' is the radius of curvature of the output half-cylinder and t is the nonlinear sample thickness. While the input and output cylinders are not required to have identical radii, using half-cylinders with very different radii will limit the maximum incidence angle that can be measured. In practice, choosing R' equal to or close to R will simplify measurements. When $R' = R$ the entire assembly forms a full cylinder centered at point A. Then, one can simply rotate the assembly 180° and use the output half-cylinder as the input and the input half-cylinder as the output, without affecting the MF measurements. Using the CMFT with an output half-cylinder that has the wrong thickness Δ_o will introduce an angle-dependent Fresnel loss at the output half-cylinder, along with a possible error in the measured MF curve. However, this error can be corrected by calculating the angle-dependent Fresnel loss at the output half-cylinder. In addition, this error can be reduced by choosing $R' \gg t$. In contrast, when using the prism-assisted technique, the Fresnel losses at the prism-air interfaces are always angle dependent. In principle, this loss is taken into account in calibration, but because of errors in the knowledge of the absolute angles of the laser and SH beams at the air-solid interfaces, the correction is never complete.

Finally, with the cylinder-assisted technique, the effective area of the laser beam at point A remains the same for all incidence angles. As a result, any error in the knowledge of this effective area is independent of incidence angle. Accurate knowledge of this effective area is important for calibration purposes. Any angle-independent error in the effective area will result in an error in the scale factor, but not in the spectral shape, of the magnitude of the FT. This error will, in turn, translate into a scale factor error in the inferred profile $d(z)$, but not in an error in the shape of this profile. In contrast, with the prism-assisted technique, the focal spot of the laser on the sample surface depends on the incidence angle θ. Furthermore, as the incidence angle is increased, the laser focal spot becomes more and more elliptical. With prisms it is therefore difficult to accurately determine the laser effective area at all angles. This inaccuracy results in an angle-dependent calibration error, which induces an error in both the scale factor *and* the shape of the inferred nonlinearity profile.

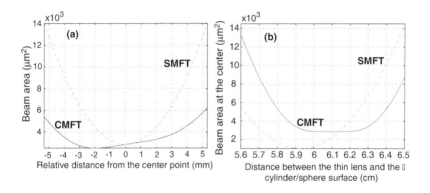

Fig. C3 (a) Dependence of the beam area on position along the z axis (see Fig. C1) calculated for CMFT and SMFT. The origin represents the center of the sphere or the cylinder. (b) The beam area at the center of the sphere/cylinder as a function of L (see Fig. C1).

As an aside, at very high incidence angles the laser beam enters the sample at grazing incidence and the SH beam exits the sample not through the output half-cylinder but through the edge of the sample. This condition occurs when $\theta > \dfrac{\pi}{2} - arctan(\dfrac{t}{R})$. To access such high angles (e.g., $87.71°$ for $t = 1$ mm and $R = 25$ mm), the edges of the sample must be polished to avoid scattering of the SH beam.

C.2 ADVANTAGES OF CMFT OVER SMFT
The cylinder-assisted technique also has important advantages over the sphere-assisted technique. A first advantage is that the effective Rayleigh range of the incident laser beam at the surface of the sample is much longer than when using half-spheres. To prove this point, we calculated the dependence of the laser beam effective area on position

along the beam propagation direction on either side of point A. This calculation, based on Gaussian beam propagation theory, was carried out for both a half-cylinder and a half-sphere. For fair comparison, the laser effective area at the sample surface was assumed to be the same in both configurations. The simulation parameters are a collimated incident laser beam at 1.064 μm with a $1/e^2$ power radius of 1.1 mm at the thin spherical lens of focal length 7.5 cm, $L = 6.1$ cm, and $R = 26.5$ mm (see Fig. C1(b)). The result of these calculations is plotted in Fig. C3(a). The abscissa origin is defined at point A. This figure shows that the Rayleigh range of the beam focused by the half-cylinder is more than twice as long as when a half-sphere is used. The reason is that with a half-cylinder, the laser beam incident on the sample surface is slightly focusing along the y direction but slightly defocusing along x. As a result, the beam area changes less rapidly in z than it does with a half-sphere, which focuses in both x and y. This property of half-cylinders is particularly important at high incidence angles, where the effective path of the laser beam through the nonlinear region becomes extremely long (e.g., a few mm) and the beam divergence starts to become significant. Even though in principle this beam divergence can be taken into account as a calibration term, there are always errors in the values of the beam parameters and the model does not faithfully reproduce reality. The use of a half-cylinder greatly reduces this undesired complication and the corresponding errors it introduces.

A second important advantage of half-cylinders over half-spheres is that the beam area is much less sensitive to focusing. Figure 3(b) plots the beam area at point A calculated versus distance L using again Gaussian beam propagation theory (the parameter values are the same as for Fig. C3(a)). With a half-cylinder the laser effective area is nearly independent of z over 3 to 4 mm, compared with only ~1 mm with a half-sphere. This independence results in easier focusing adjustment in practice.

Third, the sensitivity to lateral misalignments of the laser beam is strongly reduced when using a half-cylinder because the laser beam has to be aligned to a line along the y direction, whereas with a half-sphere it must be aligned to a single point on the surface of the half-sphere. This reduced sensitivity again makes it easier to align the input laser beam with respect to the input optics.

A final advantage of the CMFT is that one can simultaneously measure the uniformity of the sample at any given incidence angle or measure an MF curve along a line on the sample by simply translating the cylinder-sample assembly along y, both of which are impossible with half-spheres.

These combined advantages over existing techniques result in increased accuracy, easier alignment, and faster measurements, which made it possible to measure MF curves up to record incidence angles approaching $90°$, as demonstrated in the next section.

C.3 EXPERIMENTAL SET-UP AND RESULTS

The cylinder-assisted MF technique was tested with two silica samples (Infrasil, 25 x 25 x 1 mm) thermally poled at 270°C and 5 kV for 15 minutes. One of the poled samples was polished from the cathode surface down to a thickness of ~100 µm. This sample was clamped between two identical Infrasil half-cylinders of respective radius $R' = R = 26.5$ mm (see Fig. C1(b)), with index-matching gel between the sample and the half-cylinders. This configuration deviates from the ideal full cylinder illustrated in Fig. C1(b) by 100 µm, but since $R \gg 100$ µm the error introduced by this deviation is negligible. When testing the thicker sample ($t = 1$ mm), the latter was placed between an input half-cylinder of radius $R = 26.5$ mm and an output half-cylinder of $R' = R$ and $\Delta_o = 26$ mm. The deviation from the ideal full cylinder was then 500 µm, which is still acceptable since $R' \gg 500$ µm. However, one should expect the first configuration (thinner sample) to perform better in terms of the maximum achievable internal propagation angle, as demonstrated below.

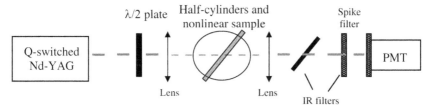

Fig. C4 Experimental set-up for Maker-fringe measurements.

Figure 4 shows the experimental set-up used for MF measurements. A $\lambda/2$ plate was used to align the state of polarization of the 1064-nm Q-switched Nd-YAG laser (~30 ns FWHM pulses, 1 kHz repetition rate) with respect to the sample (TM polarization). The cylinder-sample assembly was mounted on a rotation stage. At the output of the assembly, the beams were recollimated with a second lens and the fundamental laser signal was preferentially attenuated by ~140 dB over the second-harmonic signal with a series of IR filters and a 532-nm spike filter. The second-harmonic signal was then detected with a photomultiplier tube (PMT).

Figure 5 shows the recorded MF curves for the 0.1-mm and the 1-mm samples. Because in both measurements Δ_o differed slightly from $R' - t$, for each curve at some high incidence angle in excess of 85°, TIR sets in at the outer surface of the output half-cylinder, and above this detected angle the SH signal drops to zero. As expected from the above discussion, a larger maximum angle was obtained with the thinner sample. This maximum internal propagation angle is 89.6° (Fig. C5(b)), which is the highest value reported for an MF technique.

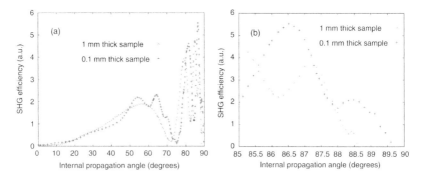

Fig. C5 (a) Experimental MF curves of thermally poled fused-silica samples measured with the test bed of Fig. C4, (b) magnified MF curves over the internal propagation angle range of 85° to 90°.

C.4 CONCLUSION

We have discussed the details of cylinder-assisted Maker fringe measurement technique that involves placing two half-cylinders against the sides of the nonlinear sample to avoid total internal reflection. This technique exhibits several important advantages over prior MF techniques, especially the possibility of achieving incidence angles extremely close to 90°, as well as increased accuracy, easier alignment, and faster measurements. These advantages are especially important for accurate characterization of thin nonlinear regions using the IFT techniques presented in Chapter 3. We experimentally demonstrated that the use of half-cylinders allows to achieve a record incidence angle of 89.6°.

REFERENCES

1. Maker, P. D., et al., "Effects of dispersion and focusing on production of optical harmonics", Phys. Rev. Lett., 8, 21, (1962)

2. D. Pureur, A. C. Liu, M. J. F. Digonnet, and G. S. Kino, "Absolute measurement of the second order nonlinearity profile in poled silica", Opt. Lett., 23, 588, (1998)

3. Quiquempois, Y., et al., "Improved method for measuring second-order non-linearity profile in poled silica", Proc. 1999 OSA Topical meeting on BGPP, Stuart, Florida, September 1999

4. A. Ozcan, M. J. F. Digonnet, and G. S. Kino, "Cylinder-assisted Maker-fringe technique," Electron. Lett. 39, 1834, (2003).

APPENDIX D: RIPPLE ANALYSIS FOR TRANSMISSION FIBER BRAGG GRATINGS

In this appendix, we derive the theoretical relationship between the unwanted magnitude ripples and the group delay ripples in a transmission fiber Bragg grating (FBG). Specifically, we prove that any transmission FBG can actually be visualized as two FBGs in series, the second one being a "hypothetical" FBG with zero physical length that represents the observed ripples in the actual FBG. We also show that the magnitude and the group delay of this "hypothetical" FBG are analytically related by the logarithmic Hilbert transform. This derivation is applicable to any transmission FBG (uniform, chirped, etc...) and supports the success of the experimental results reported in Chapter 6.

To begin, let us assume that the theoretical (i.e., designed) transmission spectrum of the FBG is given with $t_{th}(\omega) = |t_{th}(\omega)| exp(j \cdot \phi_{th}(\omega))$, where "th" stands for "theoretical". However, due to imperfections in the fabrication process, the actual transmission spectrum of the FBG becomes $t(\omega) = |t(\omega)| exp(j \cdot \phi(\omega))$, which typically has unwanted ripples both in the magnitude and the group delay spectra, as shown in Figs. 4 and 5 of Chapter 6, respectively. Without loss of generality, the actual (i.e., measured) transmission spectrum can be decomposed into.

$$t(\omega) = t_{th}(\omega) \cdot t_r(\omega) = |t_{th}(\omega)| \cdot |t_r(\omega)| \cdot exp(j \cdot (\phi_{th} + \phi_r)) \qquad (D1)$$

where "r" stands for a *hypothetical* "ripple" FBG. This decomposition is also illustrated in Fig. D1.

Since the FBG is *real*, the phase and magnitude of $t(\omega) = |t(\omega)| exp(j \cdot \phi(\omega))$ are related by the logarithmic Hilbert transform, i.e.,[1]

$$D(\omega) - D_0 = \frac{-1}{\pi} \int_{-\infty}^{\infty} \frac{\partial log(|t(\omega')|)}{\partial \omega'} \frac{d\omega'}{\omega' - \omega} \qquad (D2)$$

where $D(\omega)$ is the measured transmission group delay (with ripples), and D_0 is a constant that physically refers to the group delay caused by propagating for a distance equal to the grating length. Inserting Eq. (D1) into Eq. (D2) we get:

$$D_{th}(\omega) + D_r(\omega) - D_0 = \frac{-1}{\pi} \int_{-\infty}^{\infty} \frac{\partial log(|t_{th}(\omega')|)}{\partial \omega'} \frac{d\omega'}{\omega' - \omega} - \frac{1}{\pi} \int_{-\infty}^{\infty} \frac{\partial log(|t_r(\omega')|)}{\partial \omega'} \frac{d\omega'}{\omega' - \omega} \quad (D3)$$

where $D_{th}(\omega)$ and $D_r(\omega)$ are the group delay spectra of the theoretical (designed) FBG and the hypothetical "ripple" FBG, respectively. Since the theoretical FBG has the same physical length as the actual FBG, one can also write:

$$D_{th}(\omega) - D_0 = \frac{-1}{\pi} \int_{-\infty}^{\infty} \frac{\partial log(|t_{th}(\omega')|)}{\partial \omega'} \frac{d\omega'}{\omega' - \omega} \quad (D4)$$

Eq. (D4) also illustrates the theoretical group delay that would result if the fabricated FBG was perfect such that exactly as it was designed. Combining Eqs. (D2) and (D4) yields:

$$D_r(\omega) = -\frac{1}{\pi} \int_{-\infty}^{\infty} \frac{\partial log(|t_r(\omega')|)}{\partial \omega'} \frac{d\omega'}{\omega' - \omega} \quad (D5)$$

Eq. (D5) is an important result: it directly implies that the *hypothetical* "ripple" FBG in fact behaves like a *true* FBG, i.e., its transmission magnitude spectrum $|t_r(\omega)|$, can be computed directly from its group delay spectrum $D_r(\omega)$, and vice versa. However, the name "hypothetical" is still quite valid, since D_0 (the constant group delay) term in the left hand side of Eq. (D5) is missing, which means that the physical length of this *hypothetical* FBG is *zero*.

Therefore, we can visualize an actual measured FBG (with imperfections), as two FBGs in series; one is the theoretical (designed) FBG, and the other is the hypothetical "ripple" FBG, with zero physical length (Fig. D1).

The zero physical length argument for the hypothetical "ripple" FBG also intuitively explains the lack of multiple reflections between the two FBGs shown in Fig. D1(b), which also validates $t(\omega) = t_{th}(\omega) \cdot t_r(\omega) = \left|t_{th}(\omega)\right| \cdot \left|t_r(\omega)\right| \cdot exp(j \cdot (\phi_{th} + \phi_r))$.

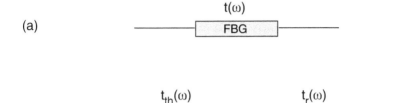

Fig. D1. (a) Illustration of a transmission FBG and (b) its equivalent component made of a series of two FBGs; the first one is the theoretical (designed) FBG and the second one is the *hypothetical* "ripple" FBG.

To summarize, in this appendix we have proved that any transmission FBG can actually be visualized as two FBGs in series, the second one of which is a hypothetical FBG with zero physical length that represents the observed ripples in the actual FBG. More importantly, we have also proven that the magnitude and the group delay of this "ripple" FBG were analytically related by the logarithmic Hilbert transform. This proof supports the success of the experimental results reported in Chapter 6.

REFERENCES

1. L. Poladian, "Group-delay reconstruction for fiber Bragg gratings in reflection and transmission", Opt. Lett. 22, 1571 (1997)

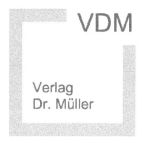

Wissenschaftlicher Buchverlag bietet

kostenfreie

Publikation

von

wissenschaftlichen Arbeiten

Diplomarbeiten, Magisterarbeiten, Master und Bachelor Theses
sowie Dissertationen, Habilitationen und wissenschaftliche Monographien

Sie verfügen über eine wissenschaftliche Abschlußarbeit zu aktuellen oder zeitlosen
Fragestellungen, die hohen inhaltlichen und formalen Ansprüchen genügt,
und haben **Interesse an einer honorarvergüteten Publikation**?

Dann senden Sie bitte erste Informationen über Ihre Arbeit per Email
an info@vdm-verlag.de. Unser Außenlektorat meldet sich umgehend bei Ihnen.

VDM Verlag Dr. Müller Aktiengesellschaft & Co. KG
Dudweiler Landstraße 125a
D - 66123 Saarbrücken

www.vdm-verlag.de

www.ingramcontent.com/pod-product-compliance
Lightning Source LLC
LaVergne TN
LVHW022304060326

832902LV00020B/3274